onto it,
nourish it.
love.

DNA MOMENTS

LINA MIRANDA

DNA Moments

Copyright © 2018 by Lina Miranda

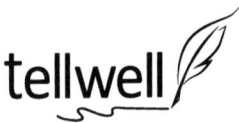

tellwell

Tellwell Talent
www.tellwell.ca

ISBN

978-0-2288-0249-5 (Hardcover)
978-0-2288-0250-1 (Paperback)
978-0-2288-0251-8 (eBook)

To the loves of my life, my husband Luch and daughter Liana,
I have found my paradise with you.

Contents

Prologue

"My scar is not so bad anymore," says Lina Braga pulling up her sweater. "I guess I've gotten used to it. Except for the keloid," she says, pointing to a slightly thicker part of the pencil-straight scar that runs from just under her breastbone to her belly button. A keloid, she explains occurs when scar tissue grows on the outer surface of a cut, instead of inside, widening the mark and creating a slight bump. "Apparently they are most common amongst African Americans, but, whatever," she says as she pulls down her top.

Lina is 22 and was diagnosed with a rare and progressive type of stomach cancer in May 2001. As we sit at the kitchen table in her parents' house and approach Cancer Awareness Month, she tries to explain what her life has been like for the past 10 months. "I used to be the weakest person. I had no backbone," Lina recalls. "It was like, instantaneously I became this strong person and had to deal with this." Lina catches herself twisting a lock of her long, shiny chestnut hair around her pinkie and smiles. She remembers making a joke about losing her hair on the day she found out about the cancer. Lina was in the bathroom she shares with her older sister, Nellie, getting ready to go out. Nellie asked her how she was going to do with her hair and Lina laughed that it didn't really matter because she was going to lose it all soon anyhow. "It was a really tasteless joke," says Nellie. "I started crying and she just laughed." Lina did not lose her hair, but she did lose 70 per cent of her stomach and about 40 pounds.

Her surgery was booked quickly and her doctor was optimistic. Results from bone scans and CAT scans had indicated that the cancer was localized. It hadn't spread. She remembers her doctor telling her that he would be opening her up and taking out anything from just the tumor, to her whole stomach. He told her she wouldn't know what she was missing until she woke up after the operation." So basically what he was saying is that if I woke up and didn't see a scar, it would be bad news because then he wouldn't have even bothered to operate on me, but if I woke up and did see a scar, it would be good news," Lina says laughing. Her good mood quickly deteriorates and her slanted green eyes lose their sparkle as she recalls the days in the hospital after surgery. Lina says those two weeks were the worst and most painful of her life, and though she appreciated the support from family and friends, she resented constantly hearing that she would be OK. "The one thing is you feel really alone in life," she says seriously. "What would piss me off is that they didn't know everything would be all right. I was the one going through the pain, I was the one with 19 staples and two tubes in me, I was the one being shot full of morphine, not them." And three days later, things only got worse. Lina's surgeon told her that the results of a biopsy he had done during surgery had come back and the cancer in her stomach had not been new and had not been localized. It had spread. The cancer had eaten its way through the layers of her stomach and reached her lymph nodes. He told her that she had been carrying the cancer inside her for maybe two years.

This catapulted Lina from being a stage one cancer patient with a 90 per cent chance of surviving, to a cancer patient halfway between stages three and four with a 20 per cent chance of surviving. "I remember that day. I had so many visitors. I just locked my door. I didn't want to see anyone," Lina stops and takes three quick breaths as her eyes fill with tears. After surgery, Lina couldn't walk properly because of her scar and couldn't even think of food without becoming nauseous. So she spent the next two weeks on the couch in her parents' living room boomeranging from periods of calm to complete breakdowns where her terror of dying became a constant companion. But, she says, she never let the friends who came to visit her know how scared she was. "If anyone ever asked how I was, I would be like, 'You know what? I'm fine.' It would be on my own time that I would cry. But you know what the funny thing is?" she says. "When I got back from surgery, I slept with my sister for three weeks," Lina looks over at Nellie and gives her a sheepish little smile. Nellie reaches over and squeezes her hand.

One month after surgery Lina began therapy. She recalls how other cancer patients receiving therapy would ask if she was there waiting for a parent. Because Lina's type of cancer is usually only found in males over the age of 50, she was always the youngest person undergoing chemotherapy. Susan, a volunteer for the Canadian Cancer Society, said that of 65,400 new cases of stomach cancer diagnosed in 2001, only 1.6 percent of the cases were female. The chemotherapy sessions would last for five days straight every month and Lina underwent six cycles of them. Her radiation was scheduled in November and lasted for 25 days, once a day. She remembers she was constantly sick and could not walk into her kitchen. The thought of food disgusted her. Lina and her mother fought constantly because she would not eat.

Lina cries again as she tells me of the one time she lost hope. It was towards the end of her radiation treatment, she says, and she weighed 90 pounds, every one of her bones stuck out and the sight of her body sickened her. She would cry every day and would not leave her bed unless it was to go to the hospital for treatment. "I came home one day, and I couldn't take it anymore," says Nellie. "She would just lay there. She smelled. I walked into her room, pulled the sheets off her and told her to go live her life. I was crying so hard, but I drew her a bubble bath, picked her up, took off her clothes and threw her in there. I wasn't going to let her give up." Lina smiles as she listens to Nellie. She says that if her sister hadn't "dumped her ass in the bath", she doesn't know what would have happened to her. She says that at that point she honestly didn't care if she died. "It's one thing to be sick and another to look sick," says Lina.

But Lina took that bath and says it was definitely a turning point for her. She realized that she had already spent so much time fighting, she wasn't about to give up so late in the game. She was done her radiation and had only one cycle of chemotherapy left. "And so, I finished it. And

I fought it. Death is a part of everyone's life," she says, smiling, "it just became a reality for me." "And now," she says, "I've gone back to school and work part time. My last scan came out clear and I took a vacation in the Caribbean to celebrate. I even wore a bikini," she says and giggles. "I guess I'm a fatalist. I believe that everything happens for a reason," she says. "And for the longest time I couldn't figure out why this had happened. But now I know it was God's message to me to enjoy every minute of my life. And you know what?" she says, "I'm 22 and love life way too much, so every day, I wake up, get out of bed and tell myself that I'm going to make it –every day."

S.M.Kranjec

Introduction

"Life is what happens when you're busy doing other things."
—John Lennon

How is it that a girl, the youngest of four kids born to immigrant parents, who was so shy and timid growing up, deathly afraid of any sort of attention and severely lacking in confidence, could end up in her thirties a successful business woman, a certified fitness instructor, and a motivational blogger and Seriously—how could this meek girl who was once so susceptible to peer pressure and obsessed with keeping up with the "Joneses" (a.k.a. the cool kids) morph herself into a strong, confident, motivated woman?

It's a question that I have often thought about and asked myself and, yes, I do have the answer to it.

Hi! I'm Lina and I'm writing this book because my life was turned upside down at the age of 21. I was diagnosed with Stage 3B stomach cancer and my odds of five-year survival were slim. Clearly, I survived, and clearly there is a story to be told. I can honestly say that I am grateful for having been faced with such a terrible and traumatic experience; I am the person I am today because of my experience fighting cancer. One of the greatest things that came out of the whole experience, aside from coming out the other side a much stronger person, is that I learned a lot about myself. I grew immensely by being able to take the time to truly reflect on myself, my character, why I am the way I am. Now, many years later, I haven't stopped reflecting; I continue to understand myself more intimately, understand why I am the person I am. I call these glimpses of self-awareness "DNA moments."

Reflecting upon the past 17 years of life post cancer, I can vividly pick out moments in my life, experiences that I have had, that have shaped me into the person I am today and continue to grow to be. We all have these moments; right now, close your eyes and just allow your brain to start recalling moments from your life. Start from childhood, work your way through high school, university, marriage and any other major milestones in your life. What do you recall? Most likely, very particular moments in your life and most likely moments that you have recalled before: repeat moments. I would argue that it's not selective memory at work here. There is more to our brain's memory recall— these moments were filed away in a special part of our brain that is intimately tied to our souls, to make us the people that we are. I am not a psychologist or claim to be an expert in psychology and must state that my claims are based solely on my beliefs. But think about it: just as unique is the fact that as these DNA moments are being lived out for the first time, we usually have no idea that they will remain with us for years to come or the importance that they will play in our future. Whether you recall these moments to learn from them, smile at them or change from them, these moments, I believe are the DNA of our future decisions in life. I don't believe that we get to choose our DNA moments; rather, I believe they have been intrinsically filed away for us and we must learn to accept them, invite them back. These moments may not always be tied to positive events in your life, but we can try to learn from them. As for the moments you love, revel in their recall!

A DNA moment is an experience or collection of experiences that get filed away into your psyche and define who you are today. They help to shape your personality, how you make decisions, and how you choose to live your life. They could be major experiences such as marriage, becoming a parent, the loss of someone we love, having to face your own mortality (such as was my case when I went through cancer), or simpler things such as making or missing a big shot at a sporting activity, or having a great or poor performance in front of people, or simply meeting someone who challenges or reinforces your beliefs.

Unlike our physical DNA which we get from our gene pool, DNA moments are collected throughout your lifetime and it is how you deal with these moments and how you use their teachings that will shape your personality and define who you are. The beauty of these moments is that although you cannot control the DNA moment itself, you can control how you perceive the moment and what you learn from it. You have the power to use these DNA moments to positively form a better version of yourself: a *you* that you can be proud of and that does not stop you from doing the things you want to do. There is something very raw about these moments, and very honest—they can expose things about you that you may not like, may regret, or may not want others to ever know about.

I have chosen to share some of my DNA moments with the world, my family, my friends, you. Every chapter of this book will make reference to one of my DNA moments from my life thus far. I will share with you the details of the moments and how I interpreted their outcomes. While I may not have all the right answers, and you may not agree with the message I am trying to convey, I can tell you that I speak from the heart, from a place of honesty and compassion. I promise to be as stripped down and open as my internal secretary allows me to be, because it is my hope that you are touched in some way, shape or form by one or all of these moments—that you may take away from my experiences something that can help you get through your next experience. "Life is what happens when you're busy doing other things" so don't get lost in the humdrum; let life happen and, for goodness sake, enjoy the ride!

Here goes nothing...

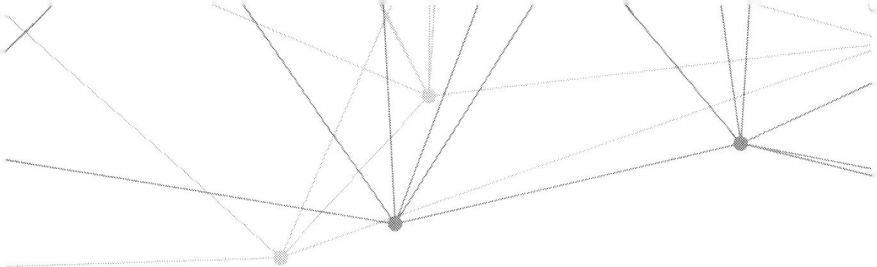

1 Mr. Handsome

Have you ever had a secret crush on someone? Come on, don't deny it. Maybe it was the barista at your favourite coffee shop, the neighbour up the street with the little cute dog or the person who stands next to you at the gym and always high-fives you at the end of class. Not all crushes have to be sexual in nature; some crushes can be more innocent, more emotional because that person just makes you feel good about yourself or that person has made such a big imprint on your life that you can't help but feel something towards him or her. It's okay to admit that you get kind of giggly or that your armpits start to sweat a little when you run into that certain someone—whatever the root of the crush, I think it's okay to have them, especially the innocent ones. Or maybe this is just my way of justifying my secret crush on Mr. Handsome. But before I get into explaining who Mr. Handsome is, yes, my husband is fully aware of my crush and he is okay with it.

Seventeen years ago I was introduced to Mr. Handsome. I did not want to meet him; in fact, I would have given anything to not have to meet him. At the time I wished he never existed and I cried at the thought of his presence in my life, but under the circumstances, I knew I had no other choice. Mr. Handsome is a surgeon, and he was my surgeon.

Mr. Handsome once told me in one of my pre-surgical visits that we are all going to die—that death should not be something that scares one person more than another, that the only difference between me and most people was that my dying had become a reality for me.

So how did this become my reality?

Let's rewind two years prior to my diagnosis. I was your typical first-year university student living in a dorm, doing the typical things that most 18-year-olds do and, of course, feeling overwhelmed with my course load. First-year science at the University of Toronto was stressful to say the least.

It was at this time that I remember experiencing my first symptoms, symptoms such as acid reflux that I was told by my family doctor were due to stress. First year came and went and the symptoms grew worse. I decided to move back home for the remainder of my degree—dorm life was great and I had made many wonderful friends and memories, but the cost to live on campus was prohibitive, especially considering the fact that I lived only 30 minutes from the downtown campus and not even 15 minutes from a satellite campus. Looking back, being close to home may have been my saving grace; it kept my relationship with my then-boyfriend afloat. During the first half of my second year, I made multiple visits to my family doctor, went through courses of PPI meds (for reducing stomach acid), tested positive for and received treatment for an *H.pylori* ulcer, and still my symptoms worsened. Worsened to the point that I admitted myself to the emergency room numerous times for severe burning pain in my stomach, desperately asking for morphine to take me out of my misery and drinking crazy amounts of milk to soothe my stomach—worsened to the point that I knew something was wrong.

The night of my last visit to the emergency room prior to being diagnosed was one of those moments for me: a DNA moment. I had woken up early in the morning; it must have been around 2:00 a.m. or so and I was in excruciating pain. The pain felt like someone had rolled up a cloth towel, soaked it in gasoline and then lit it on fire inside my stomach. I hemmed and hawed about waking my up my father to take me to the hospital; I knew that the IV of Demerol would make me feel better but I just did not have the energy to go back and yet again be told to go home 12 hours later. Being that it was just after two in the morning, I opted to call my boyfriend to complain about the pain that I was in. He should have been on his way home from his shift at the bar where he was working; instead, he had finished work and was having a drink with a friend at a bar just down the street from his. Being very young and somewhat immature, I asked who his friend was and he said, "Just an old friend," but his vagueness sparked a little insecurity in me so I continued to pry until he finally told me that it was an old girlfriend who had come by his work to say hi and that they had decided to go for a drink afterwards. Knowing that nothing was really going on aside from him having a drink with an old friend, I still felt the need to be catty and rather than hang up, tell him goodnight and crawl into a fetal position in my bed, I told him that he needed to leave right away so he could drive me to the hospital. (I actually wanted nothing to do with the hospital, but I wanted even less to do with my boyfriend having drinks with another girl as I lay awake in pain. Without hesitating, he said of course and just as quickly hung up the phone and left his old friend to finish her beer by herself.

I was asked by the ER physician if I had ever been scoped; he thought that someone my age should not be experiencing such severe stomach pain resulting in repeat emergency room visits unless there was something going on. His suspicions were nothing serious—he thought that perhaps I had a perforated ulcer. Knowing my age would put me at the bottom of a very long wait list for an endoscopy if he sent me home, he asked if he could admit me to the hospital so that I could get priority and be seen by a gastroenterologist the next day. My answer was yes, especially since I had plans to go backpacking with my best friend and our boyfriends in Europe next month. I was eager to find out what the heck was wrong with me and hopefully get my ulcer fixed so that I would be in tip-top shape for conquering Europe. This was to be my first trip on my own. I had bamboozled my parents into agreeing to let me travel around Europe with my best friend Stef. The story I told them was that Stef and I would travel through Europe together for a few weeks, just us girls, before making our way to Portugal where we would meet up with our boyfriends (her boyfriend was my boyfriend's best friend) and my boyfriend's family at his summer home. Knowing that there would be parental supervision, my parents were okay with the fact that I would be on vacation with my boyfriend—yes, they were those kinds of parents. The kind that didn't allow me to stay overnight with anyone who had a Y chromosome. Embarrassingly, I can admit that I had the strictest, most naïve Portuguese parents ever. Actually thinking back, I don't think they were all that naïve; I think they just chose to stay in their little bubble and ignore what may happen outside of it. The *real* plan for our trip was that the four of us would travel together throughout Europe, and—not completely lying to my parents—we would indeed end up in Portugal at my boyfriend's parents' summer house. Throughout a lot of my teens and early twenties, I was a master of omission of facts. Some may call it lying, but I call it selective truth-telling. The short of it was that this Europe trip meant more to me on so many different levels than just any regular summer vacation. So, YES, admit me to the freaking hospital and fix my stomach so that I may go off to discover Europe with my bestie and my Y-chromosome companion!

After being released from the hospital, I went on with my everyday life, thinking nothing at all about my scope or its results. I continued to waitress at a café until the early morning hours most nights and would sleep in to the early afternoon most days. It was probably one week after my discharge that my father mentioned to me that a doctor from the hospital had tried calling a couple of times that week, wanting to speak with me, but I was either working or not home and he didn't leave a message, simply saying that he would continue to try calling. On his third attempt he reached me.

I will never forget picking up the phone in my bedroom and hearing the doctor on the other line ask me if I was sitting down. It was in that moment that my life changed—my life as I knew it, all of my plans, from what I was going to do that day to my trip next month, it all changed. I remember everything about that moment. I remember wearing grey cotton drawstring shorts with a navy blue University of Toronto sweatshirt. I remember that my hair was up in a bun sitting high on my head. My bed was unmade; the navy blue comforter with green and purple details lay crumpled at the foot of the mattress. I had just woken up and was standing at my closet door staring aimlessly at my clothes, wondering what I should pack for my trip. More specifically, I was thinking to myself how the heck am I going to fit all of my necessities for more than a month of travel into the one purple backpack that I had just purchased for my trip? It was a 50-litre backpack, a really nice one. I remember smiling every time I saw it there on my floor, smiling with the knowledge that it would soon be strapped to my back as I embarked on what should have been the best time of my life. I remember thinking to myself, "Why the heck is he asking if I'm sitting down?" But as pedantic as a selective-truth-telling young adult, I sat on my bed, staring at the backpack which was laid out beautifully in front of my closet, and that is when I heard the word for the first time: tumor. And then, "malignant." It was not bad enough to hear those words, but to hear the uncertainty in a physician's voice as he said them was a moment that will forever be engrained in my memory. I frantically reached over to my desk and moved around some textbooks in search of a piece of paper and a pen and began to write down the dates for upcoming scans that had been booked for me—booked to determine the extent of my cancer and its spread, or hopefully lack of.

Many people try to pinpoint times in their lives that they can say were significant ones, the ultimate DNA moments, if you will. Moments that allowed them to take one path vs. another at a fork in the road, a fork that they may not have even known they were travelling towards. For me, this was that moment, the moment that weak Lina became strong Lina—the Lina that would have to learn to not give up and have faith that she could do anything that she put her mind to, could jump over any hurdle, could say to herself—"Yes, you can"—and actually believe her own words.

As I sat on my bed, staring at the purple backpack, listening to the sound of silence on the other end of the phone, I pressed the end button, took a deep breath, wiped the tears from my eyes and stood up. Walking out of my bedroom, down the spiral staircase holding on to the banister for strength, hanging on for hope and courage to find the words that I would have to say in a moment's time, I slowly made my way downstairs and found my mom and dad in the kitchen. Deep breaths. Chest proud, no tears, I looked them in the eyes and said, "Mom, Dad, I have cancer."

The next two weeks were consumed with doctor's appointments and scans. Up until these scans, all the doctors knew, all I was told, was that I had a tumor in the posterior bottom portion of my stomach measuring approximately three to four centimetres. With no definite confirmation of its confinement or spread, and whether it had affected any of my other organs, I could only hope for the best but prepare myself for the worst. Fortunately, the scans showed no signs of metastasis, and so I was confirmed for surgery in two weeks.

I'll never forget meeting Mr. Handsome for the first time. I sat in his small office that was no bigger than a walk-in closet, squished between my entourage of support at the time: my boyfriend, his mother, his father, my father, my sister and I believe one of my two brothers. Being Portuguese and all, we never travel light or do much on our own; it's usually a family affair. The room was nothing special: an examining table, which at the moment was a makeshift bench for my entourage, a chair which I sat on and a stool where Mr. Handsome would soon sit. The walls were covered with various anatomical posters; the one of particular interest to me depicted a stomach and intestines, slightly raised off the paper, giving it a dimensional look. Mr. Handsome opened the door to the small room and, probably surprised by the number of people that could fit inside, sat down on his stool and smiled. His eyes sparkled and his smile warmed my anxious heart.

"So, I'm going to go in laparoscopically first and look around. If it is inoperable, I won't go on with the surgery. Worst-case scenario—you wake up without a scar, best case scenario, you wake up with a scar and part of your stomach. My intent is to salvage as much of the upper portion of the stomach as I can to be able to connect to the intestine."

I know—I was thinking the exact same thing that you're thinking right now. No stomach? How the heck would I eat? Apparently people can survive without a stomach and live to be healthy and old individuals. Naturally, he explained it would take some adjustment, and my feeding and eating habits would need to change, but essentially he said nothing that would stop me from doing the things that I desired in life. I could even still have children, which was actually one of the first questions out of my mouth: "Can I carry a healthy baby to term without a stomach?"

Sensing what must have been the sheer look of panic and fright in my eyes, Mr. Handsome put his hand on my knee, looked me in the eyes and said, "Death is something that will happen to us all— it can happen to me tomorrow crossing the street— but the difference between you and me and the rest of us in here in this room is that death has been made a *conscious* reality for you, whereas for us it's not something that we are forced to have to deal with in our everyday reality." He was right—so much more right than I think he knew he was. What he told me that day, on our first encounter, in that small room covered with anatomical posters, is the essence, the foundation for how I hope to live the rest of my life. Death *is* going to happen, you and I will die. What we must do is remember to live each day, make every decision keeping in mind that we are not immortal and that one day we will face our death, our end to this gift of life on earth, and at that time we must have no regrets. To not have regrets is to ensure that we take chances, to believe that we can leap over the hurdles placed in front of us and do the unthinkable, to believe in ourselves, to say, "Yes, I can," and believe what you've said.

Two weeks later, eight-and-a-half hours after being wheeled off to surgery, with an ever-growing entourage that now included 20-plus family members and friends, I woke up. Waking up after such a long surgery I had a sense of panic as I opened my eyes; it didn't take long before I tried to move my cover off me to look for a scar. My surgical nurse tried to calm me down, gently placing her hands on mine and saying, "Sweetie, don't worry.

You're okay, the surgery went well." Not knowing if her definition of "well" included waking up with a scar, I asked her if there was a scar, and with a smile on her face she answered, "Yes." If I was not so high on meds, I think I would have jumped up out of my bed and done a cart-wheel (that is of course if I could do a cartwheel—to this day I still have not figured out how, I have a strange fear of being upside down).

The next day I woke up feeling less groggy and was ready to do a recon of my body. There was one large dress-ing stemming from my bra line down to my naval. There were two drainage tubes coming out of each side of my lower abdomen, a catheter bag and an NG tube (a suction tube that is placed in the nose to help pump liquids from the stomach). Additionally, there was a morphine pump that was controlling the amount of morphine being dripped into my body via my epidural. Above me was a triangular apparatus that I later learned was for me to use to try and prop myself up on the mattress; as I had been cut right through my abdominal wall, I would have little to no mid-section strength for quite some time as I recovered.

As the days passed, I was slowly weaned off of my con-stant morphine drip and given a pump that would only allow a certain amount of drug when needed. My catheter was removed and I was encouraged to start walking and going to the washroom on my own. Going to the bathroom was quite the ordeal; I would have to start prepping myself a solid 15 minutes before really having to go. Remember, no abdominal strength to get up from bed, tubes sticking out of me and an IV rack and morphine pump that needed to come along with me. Making it to the toilet in time was such a win for me—sad how my goals had changed in such a short amount of time from conquering Europe on my own to making it to the bathroom in time without peeing on the floor. The days went by, and with each passing day I was able to get rid of a few more tubes and eventually I was tube-free.

It was time for another visit from Mr. Handsome. In his dreamy way, he sat down on my bedside, smiled and put his hand on mine, then asked if I wanted the good news or the bad news first. I asked for the good news first; let the good lessen the blow of the bad. The good news was that he had successfully removed the entire tumour with excellent margins; there was no tumour left inside my stomach. The bad news was that the pathology report of my surrounding lymph nodes had tested positive for a percentage that staged my cancer at a 3B, giving me a five-year survival rate of only 20%. Instant tears welled up in my eyes as I listened to him tell me that I would have to endure chemotherapy and radiation in an attempt to fight this upcoming battle for my survival.

And so, there you have it: just when you think life has thrown its wildest curveball at you, you're struck by another one. They say (not really sure who they are) but they say that what doesn't kill you will make you stronger—isn't that the truth? I was not going to let this cancer kill me, so my cancer could only make me stronger.

Six months later, after having endured six rounds of chemotherapy, 25 days of radiation, and having lost 40 pounds, bringing me down to a sickly 90 pounds, I had done all that I could do. Now it was up to me to believe that I would beat the odds, that I would be that one in five who survived five years, because in my eyes, there was no other option: I was not done living. I wanted to graduate university, I wanted to get married and have a family. I wanted to be a mom.

Being faced with a challenge, whether personal or professional in nature, can be daunting and overwhelming at first. It can be difficult to see the light at the end of the tunnel and understand how it is that you will get there, or even if you will. The belief that you will get there is definitely a necessity because without it, you are setting yourself up for failure. But belief is not everything; you also need a plan. Whether you are a planner or not, some things in life require some sort of formal structure, as opposed to a "cross your fingers and hope for the best" mentality. Plans can vary in complexity, from something as simple as having a virtual map in your mind to coming up with a formal, indexed document, but whatever your plan looks like, I do believe that having one is the key to success and here is why.

The process of creating a plan (regardless of its complexity) allows you to fully understand the challenge or task at hand. It forces you to dissect the situation and look at all the aspects of it to gain insight into what the various obstacles, challenges, or positive outcomes may be ahead of time. The process of creating the plan will undoubtedly help you become not only more comfortable with the challenge, but it will help guide you along your journey. When I was faced with the biggest challenge of my life— beating the odds and surviving cancer—I was lost at first. I had no idea how I was going to survive, but I knew that

I needed some sort of plan because sitting back and hoping for the best was not going to be enough.

My plan was never a formal one, nor was it a linear one, but it was one that helped me find the light. The first step in my plan was to do research. I googled everything and anything that had the words stomach and/or cancer in the same document. I wanted to know everything that there was to know about my situation—the good the bad and the ugly. I wanted to be prepared for everything that may or may not happen with my recovery, my treatments and how others had overcome their battles. In the upcoming chapters I will share with you the aspects of my plan for survival—many of them I now classify as a being DNA moments, moments that undoubtedly shaped me into the person I am today, post-cancer Lina.

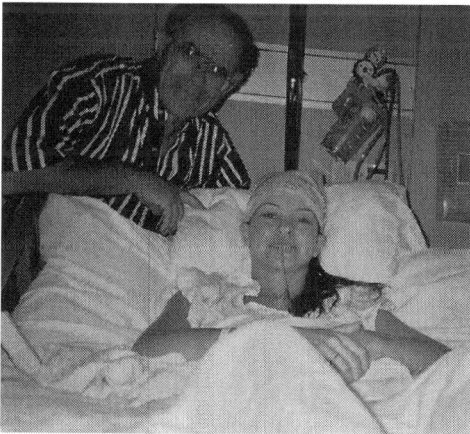

My dad and I a week after my surgery

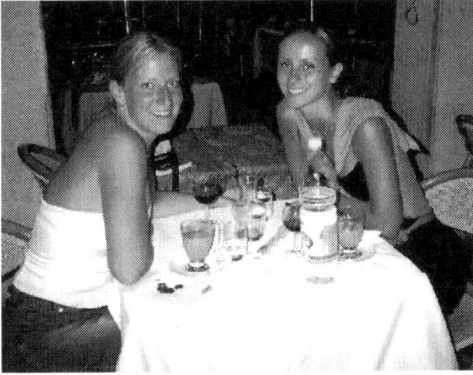

My best friend Stef and I having dinner in
Italy. One year after my diagnosis.

2 Faith and Pac-Mans

Being raised by very Catholic parents, I grew up with a strong religious influence. I had the saint statue and rosary sanctuary in the formal dining room of my childhood home—the same sanctuary that every other Portuguese home also housed in its plastic-wrapped French provincial–style dining and living room. We had crucifixes in all of the bedrooms and over each door at every entrance to the house. Every Sunday we all got dressed in our finest for Sunday mass; my father would squeeze me, the youngest, my sister and two brothers into the back of his Volare (a 1970s-style station wagon with wood panelling—yes, we rode in style) with my mom in the front, and drive us to mass, where we would be the first ones to arrive. We sat in the same pew on the same side of the same row every single week. In front of us and behind us were always the same families, dressed in their Sunday best, as well. This exact same ritual took place every week; as the years went by, my oldest brother eventually got his driver's licence and would drive himself to the later mass, then my next oldest brother did the same, and four years after that, my sister got her licence and she, too, like our brothers would soon drive the two of us to the later mass every Sunday. As

I'm sure you've guessed by now, rather than go to the later mass, we played hooky and went to the nearby coffee shop for an hour and drank coffee with our other Portuguese friends who were also driving themselves to the later mass. Eventually, I got my licence and my parents were officially on their own to continue with their Sunday routine of sitting in the same pew of the same row on the same side of the church that they had for many years.

Having grown up with parents who had such a deeply rooted faith in their religion, you would think that I would have felt the same way, but the truth of the matter was that I was young and had little reason to pay much attention to matters of faith or religion. That is, of course, until the weeks leading up to June 21st, the date of my surgery. I remember the Sunday after I was diagnosed and just a few short weeks before my surgery, my parents told me that they had spoken to the priest and had added my name to the list of the sick to be prayed for during mass. Talk about making it official. When they say your name out loud in church and ask for everyone to pray for you, you are officially sick, and of course, the list of the sick always comes just before the list of those "no longer with us." As a sick person hearing your name out loud, you can't help but ask yourself, "Am I eventually going to be on the next list?" Many months would pass before I would have enough strength to go back to church, but in those months that I was not physically able get there, my faith grew in leaps and bounds.

I don't think I have ever shared with anyone (not even my husband), how my faith developed while I was sick. I don't actually know why I've never shared this before—it's been my little secret up until now—but in the interest of transparency and openness, here goes nothing.

There were many nights that I would go to bed and feel so utterly alone and afraid. I suppose I never shared with anyone how afraid I was because I didn't want anyone to think of me as being weak. The nights, especially in the beginning soon after my surgery and before my treatment, I was afraid to fall asleep because I was afraid that I would not wake up. In fact, I actually slept with my sister in her bed for two weeks after my release from the hospital. She believed it was because I had troubles getting in and out of bed due to my surgery and that it was best if I had someone by my side to help me during the night in case I needed to get up to go to the bathroom. Yes, I did need the physical help, but more than that, what I needed the most was the company someone next to me while I was falling asleep so I wouldn't be left alone to think and be afraid.

Once I had graduated to sleeping in my own room again, I spent many nights fighting sleep and trying to stay awake. Oftentimes, I would look for things to distract me; when nothing on TV appealed to me, I would start rummaging through my bedside tables. One night, I remember looking through one of my night-table drawers and discovering a Bible in one of them. I believe my mother had placed Bibles in all of my siblings' bedside tables. This Bible that I had hidden deep in my drawer and never paid any attention to would turn out to be my saving grace. Who would have thought that I would find so much strength from it? Sure as heck not me. My first night with the Bible, I think I just sat and looked at it. I remember feeling a little torn. I didn't want to be the type of person who only turned to God when it was convenient for them and because now, all of a sudden, I had a reason to. But that's not what I did. Instead, I turned to the glossary and searched under *M* for "Miracles," and metaphorically speaking, the gates to Heaven opened and the angels sang, and my faith was born. And so, every night for many weeks, I had my own little secret affair with the Bible. I folded over the pages of all of the passages that had any mention of a miracle in it. The ones with a miracle involving the sick were really special ones and they often received a half-page fold rather than just a corner fold. I found so much strength in reading these passages, I began to have faith that miracles could happen and the more I read these passages, the more I believed that I would be okay.

Having the belief that I would be okay was not enough to satisfy my body's need for sleep, though, and I needed more to help protect against the possibility of not waking up. It was time to take action in my own mind, which brings us to Secret #2 and one of the elements of my survival plan: my nightly encounters with Pac-Mans.

As I had mentioned previously, part of my plan to survive was to research the heck of what I was dealing with and read about other patients' stories. In my research, I had come across an article about a little boy who had a brain tumour and was given only months to live. In a follow-up visit to the hospital, the doctors were shocked to see that his tumour had shrunk since his last visit. Without being able to explain it any other way, the doctors told the boy's mother that a miracle had happened and that his tumour had shrunk in size. The young boy then said, "No, Mommy, it wasn't a miracle—it was the fighters." This little boy explained that every night before he fell asleep, he would close his eye and imagine little Pac-Mans eating away at his brain tumour.

Miracles or Pac-Mans...Why choose? So I didn't—I chose both. Every night I would read about biblical miracles and after placing my secret Bible back in its drawer hidden under a mess of papers, I would lie on my back, close my eyes and fall asleep to little cartoon-like creatures eating away at any remaining cancer cells in my stomach and greater abdominal area. Night time was no longer such a scary time for me, or a lonely time; I had found comfort in my miracles and my imaginary friends. Whether this part of my plan would work or not, I had found the solace I needed to get through the nights.

Undoubtedly, we have all had time when we've felt utterly alone and like there is no one else in the world that understands what we are going through. Moments when, even though people around us tell us that we will be okay, we can't help but question whether or not we will be. It's in these moments that we need to remember to keep an open mind to the things around us, tangible or not, that can help get us through such difficult times. Self doubt can start to take a wrong turn down positive lane with you at the driver's seat. In my case, what got me over my sense of fear was the plan that I had constructed for myself to get through the nights. My plan involved reinforcing my belief that I would be okay by finding strength in my newly born faith and training my brain to fight off rogue cells. Even if imagining Pac-mans eating away at my rogue cancer cells was completely ridiculous, at least it provided me with the comfort to fall asleep on my own at the time when I felt my weakest and most lonely; it gave me the strength to get through the night and wake up to a new day.

My faith had a religious foundation, but not all faith has a religious footing to it. In fact, I would argue that the word "faith" could be easily interchanged with the word "belief." Having faith or belief is so fundamental to our existence. I believe that faith is to our survival like fuel is to a car; without faith, we are simply stalled vehicles, revving our engines with no hope of moving forward. Without believing that we can or that we will, we can't and we won't. So what is the secret, then? How do we get rid of all of the self-doubt that we sometimes feel? Why is it that some people walk around like they have all the confidence in the world and others hide under a shell of doubt? There really is no true answer to this, but here is the good news… with practice, we can all become shareholders in the word "Believe", and what's even more awesome is that the more we believe, the more we will become. If there is one thing that I have learned from my experiences it is that we must first be vulnerable enough to accept our weaknesses and our fears. It is not until you know what is stopping you from doing what you want to do that you can begin to work on finding a solution. It was very difficult for me to admit to myself that I was afraid of death because admitting it made it so much more real. Admitting to myself that I was afraid to be alone at night and fall asleep because I was not sure if I would wake up was scary! But once I had accepted my fears and my doubts, I was able to find solace. For me, solace was hiding in a religion that I had mostly ignored in previous years and in my imaginary animated friends. Whatever your belief is rooted in, you must remember to be open to finding it, and when you do find it, you will become so strong and able to take on any challenge that life throws at you.

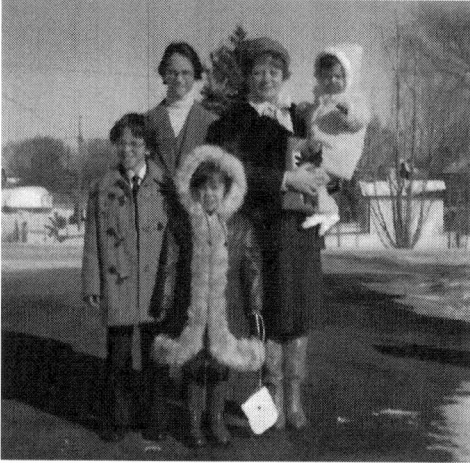

My family and I (the little one in my mom's arms) in our Sunday best on our way to church.

3 Nature vs. Nurture

As a science major and someone who has taken numerous courses in human biology and psychology, you would think that I would be closer to solidifying my opinion on this age-old question, Nature Or Nurture?; but, the truth is, I'm not. I'm still sitting on the fence, one leg hanging off each side of this debate. If I were to base the answer solely on my life and my experiences, then that would explain my choice of seat.

Through my teen years and into my early twenties, pre-cancer Lina was weak, not simply physically, but emotionally and mentally weak. I'm sure if my friends and family at the time had been interviewed, they all would have reported that they did not believe that I would have the strength to get through what I went through.

My parents were modest immigrants living in a suburb of Toronto, Ontario, Canada, raising a family of four children on one income. My parents never encouraged me the way I remember some of my friends' parents encouraged them to do things—to join the basketball team, to become an astronaut, to strive for the moon and shoot for the stars. My parents were just parents; they put food on the table and ensured we had a safe roof over our heads. Their nurturing was not of the sort that would provide me with the catalyst to become a strong-willed, confident women; on the contrary, I believe that the way I was raised instilled in me my ever-so annoying self-confidence issues that I continue to harbour to this day. Please, don't get me wrong; I love my mom and my dad, may he rest in peace, but the truth is they did nothing for my confidence growing up. Why do I blame them, you ask? Why not debate that nature is responsible for the annoying aspects of my personality, not my parents? To that I say, because I evolved—I was able to and continue to evolve. I have become post- cancer Lina, the Lina who believes that she can reach for the moon and shoot for the stars. Post-cancer Lina was always there; she just needed to be nurtured to become who she is. The nurturing that got me to who I am today is embedded in the experiences that I faced at 21, fighting for my life, facing the reality of my death. The fact of the matter is that we all have it in us—we all have the ability to do great things and become great people whatever that may be to you. We have different definitions of greatness; the point is that we can do it, but you have to believe in yourself first. Think of life as a blank canvas: you, alone, are the artist, the paint, the paintbrush. You control what masterpiece you will become. Yes, art is subjective and its beauty lies in the eyes of the beholder, and that is exactly the point. You control your canvas and you must see the work in progress as a masterpiece first and foremost before anyone else.

You control your emotions, your beliefs, your choices and your life. Remember, "Life is what happens when you are busy doing other things" John Lennon said, so don't get caught up on what you are going to paint or what brush to use, whether to use oil or acrylic—just paint. Take your leaps of faith, step outside of your comfort zone, live with no regrets, believe that you can and you will. The only thing stopping you from doing anything is yourself.

So where does science fit into this, then? There is published research showing that our brains at a young age are wired into pathways that are responsible for, or which explain, our adult personalities. This same research also shows that with time and training we can change these pathways and alter how our brain is hardwired. We can do this by forcing ourselves to live through experiences that force our brain to adapt to various situations and therefore become more adaptable to new environments. There is a reason why life coaches and motivational speakers are an industry that is booming—there is a demand for support in individual development and the demand is increasingly rising. I get it, though; not everyone is comfortable admitting that they need help, nor do most people even believe that they need it. It takes a lot for a person to have an honest look at themselves and be truthful about their current state. Prior to my illness, I admit that I thought I was just fine, superficially—I had a job, a boyfriend, no major issues and I enrolled in a great university where I had many friends. However, beneath the surface, if I was truly honest with myself, I was a very insecure, shy and timid person. Someone who, although I got good grades, never thought I was smart enough; although I always had guys asking for my phone number, never thought I was pretty enough. I was consumed with doubt and insecurities, and if I am being honest with myself now, I do attribute many of those feelings to my upbringing. We are who we are, and I'm sure my parents did the best they could do raising us, and I'm sure that their parenting style mirrored their upbringing, as well. What matters most for me, and what I hope to convey to you, is that recognizing your limitations and taking the step towards working to become the best *you* that you can be is what really matters.

Pre-cancer Lina vs. post-cancer Lina. The experience for me of going through something so life-altering forced me to become a stronger person; it forced me to learn how to deal with certain emotions and fears that I probably would not have had to deal with otherwise. One of my greatest fears was being up in front of people; I hated having any sort of attention drawn to me and the idea of having to do a presentation in front of people or do any sort of public speaking horrified me. I could only imagine all the terrible things that people would say about me. All of these thoughts, negative and unfounded, were simply fictitious mind-talk that my fear created. In a later chapter I will touch on overcoming this fear in my quest to pursue a dream of mine, and I will speak to how it was through my new-found love for fitness (a love that I stumbled across as a means to survive my cancer) that allowed me to conquer this fear.

My experience being diagnosed with cancer taught me that I was capable of making it through unthinkably difficult life circumstances. It allowed me to truly reflect upon myself and be honest with who I was and who I wanted to become. Clearly, I am not suggesting that everyone should be diagnosed with a terminal illness to make them a stronger person, but what I am suggesting is that, through experiences, you should allow yourself to be open to honest introspection and know that you do have the ability to change and create new pathways for yourself.

Having met my husband a year almost to the date of my surgery was definitely a DNA moment for me. Having him in my life has been the positive, motivational, loving influence that has provided me with a safe place to grow and thrive. Without a doubt, Luch (Luciano, although I've only ever called him that once, and it was during our wedding vows) has been the catalyst for me fulfilling many of my goals, encouraging me to not back down and reminding me of the person I am today: capable, willing and determined. He often says that I am the one who gives him the courage to take on wildly ambitious goals and to live his life to the fullest, so I guess we both help each other in this way.

We met on June 20, 2002. At first glance, I thought he was a five-foot-nothing, short Spanish guy. He thought I was a typical snobby, pretty girl. We were both wrong and had both made terrible assumptions. Both assumptions were formed based on the fact that I was pretty doped up on pain meds, although he was unaware of that at the time.

The night prior to our "meet cute"—a term given to fictional scenes in a movie when two romantic leads meet for the first time—I had been co-hosting my sister's and future brother-in-law's Jack and Jill party. The party took place at my future brother-in-law's brother's house. The house was full; there was loud music and drinks flowing. Sometime around 1:00 a.m., I was walking through the backyard to get to the neighbours' yard so that I could get some more ice, as our bartender (who I might add was my ex-boyfriend) was running out. Somehow, I managed to loose my footing on some uneven grass, twisted my foot and went crashing down. Some time had passed before anyone noticed that I was crawling back into the house unable to put any pressure on my foot. Luckily, my best friend Stef had not been drinking (she had to be able to drive us both back to my house bright and early the next day where one of her friends was going to pick us up to drive to a beach volleyball tournament), so she and I went straight to the hospital to get my ankle looked at.

The party was taking place in a smaller town about an hour west of the city; this smaller town came with a smaller hospital that had no X-ray techs working the night shift, so we had to make our way to the larger hospital that was actually much closer to my house. By now, it was probably 3:00 a.m. and our ride was coming to get us at 6:00 a.m for the volleyball tournament, which was taking place a two hours east of the city.

The wait at the second hospital was very long, so I made the executive decision to buy some crutches and a tensor bandage and go enjoy the beach for the day and come back that night to get my ankle looked at. It was either wait at the hospital in pain or wait on a beach in pain, so I chose the latter. Stef and I grabbed some McDonald's breakfast to go and made our way to my place. On the ride over, Stef called Bobby, her friend who was coming to get us, to explain that I may or may not have a broken ankle and was on crutches and some old painkillers that I had found in the medicine cabinet. His response was "Not a problem— I'll bring some frozen peas and a pillow to elevate her foot." Bobby, who is actually Luch's best friend, had met Stef a few weeks back for the first time in almost 10 years. They were childhood friends, both their families belonged to the same Slovenian cultural group, but the two had lost touch once they both stopped participating in the cultural dancing competitions. What I did not realize was that Bobby had given Luch the heads-up that a green-eyed, brown-haired girl (me) was coming to the tournament on the weekend to watch. Bobby, knowing Luch's preference in girls, thought that Luch and I would make a great couple.

When Luch first arrived, I was lying down on the sand on a towel, groggy from my pain meds and in a lot of pain. He had not noticed my crutches nearby, nor my very swollen foot. He tried making conversation with me, but I wanted nothing to do with anything but sleeping off the pain. Hence, his first assumption of me was that I was snobby, and my first impression of him only being five feet tall was the meds talking.

Once Luch learned what had happened to me, he was quite the gentleman, bringing me ice for my foot and piggybacking me around the beach. It turned out that he was six feet tall, strikingly handsome and probably one of the best things that ever happened to me.

The decision I made that day in the hospital to go off to the beach regardless of the uncertain state of my ankle may have been a somewhat reckless one, but it was one of the best decisions of my life. I know for sure the old Lina (pre-cancer Lina) would have waited in the ER for hours and not have gone off to the beach with a swollen foot, but the new Lina, well, she knew that there was no grave danger in her prolonging the X-ray, so she chose the less safe of the two options and, as a result, ended up having one of her most memorable DNA moments.

It turned out that my ankle was badly sprained; an air-cast was required for a couple of weeks, but it was nothing serious. Luch and I started dating and, just over a year later, we were engaged. Then, just over a year after that we were married. We have been married almost 13 years now, and not a day goes by that I don't feel blessed to get to share my life with him. He provides for me an environment that allows me to thrive, allows me to continue to nurture post-cancer Lina and not allow the insecurities of pre-cancer Lina to sneak their way back.

For me, my current nurture, my environment, my surroundings, who I choose to have in my life and what I choose to do with my life, continues to be the driving force behind bringing out the best and dulling the worst of my nature.

4 The Craziness of Growing up

I suppose that one good thing about being a child is the naivety that children possess. Growing up, I just assumed that my mom's crazy shenanigans were normal, or at least that's what I told myself because I didn't know any better. Now, as a mature adult, I can reflect back on my childhood and make more sense of the crazy environment that we lived in. The crazy was not all the time, but it when it was on, it was on.

My mother met my father when she was 16 in the little town that she grew up in on one of the Portuguese islands. In those days, dating was nothing like it is today; men would have to court the women and they could only be together if chaperoned. My mother would stand outside on the second-floor balcony of her home and speak to my father on the street level below. My father was older than my mother by nine years, which at that time was a big deal. My great-grandfather, who was like a father to my mother (her father had passed away when she was only four), did not like the idea of my father trying to court his precious little girl. As luck would have it for my great-grandfather, my father decided to move to Canada to work on the Canadian Pacific Railway. Back in the '50s the CPR was calling men from Europe over to Canada to help build the railway. Although my father had left Portugal, he continued to court my mother via letters. And it was pretty much through a letter that he proposed to her and they planned their wedding. After many years, my father returned to the island to marry my mother and bring her back with him to Canada. My mother essentially married a stranger and then travelled over the Atlantic Ocean to a new country—a place where she knew no one, did not speak the language and only had my father to depend on. When I think about the courage that it must have taken her to do so, I'm impressed. I don't know if I could have done it.

Shortly after they settled into their tiny little flat in a tiny little town called Streetsville, which at the time was surrounded by farms and built around one main street that ran through the town, my oldest brother was born. Four years after, my second oldest brother was born and not only was the family growing, the town was growing, too. My parents moved the family out of the flat and into a house. My brothers were probably around nine and five when things started to happen with my mom. Her neighbour at the time started to stalk her. Little things at first—crank calls and peeping through the windows—turned into bigger things: crude comments over the phone and more explicit stares. This ongoing torment that my mother experienced triggered something within her that landed her in a mental ward. Back in the late '70s, electric shock therapy was a standard therapy for mental patients and my mother has horrible memories of this being done to her. She spent over three months at the local hospital in the mental ward, while my brothers spent those months with a family member who was helping my father juggle work, visits to the hospital and two young boys.

My mother, I'm told was never the same afterwards. She did go on to have two more children, myself being the youngest. It's actually quite sad, but I don't remember much of the good stuff: the fun times or family vacations that we took. I know we took them because I see us as a family in the pictures from our vacations, but I don't remember them. What I do remember is the crazy times, the times that my mom would loose her shit and spiral into an "episode." I remember all too often our family doctor having to make a house call to sedate my mother because my father could no longer control her. Knowing what I know now about mental illness, I know it was not her fault for being the way she was, but at the time, it was really tough to go through.

One memory that I have, one of the DNA moments that I wish I did not recall, happened when I was no more than six or seven. I had been playing in my mom's bedroom and came across her bottles of nail polish and decided that I wanted to paint my nails. In trying to get the nail polish remover bottle open, I accidently spilled some on my mother's dresser and it ate away at the varnish, leaving a discoloured patch. I was so afraid of what my mother was going to do to me that I remember crying and running for the bathroom; I locked myself in the bathroom in fear of my mother. The details are a little blurry, but the next thing I remember is my mother somehow getting me out of the bathroom and handing me a plastic grocery bag while yelling at me to pack my clothes and get out of the house. She kicked me out of the house! I vividly recall balling my eyes out and walking down the driveway, feeling so ashamed of myself and so unloved; I was so afraid and alone. And that is the last of my memory. I can't recall how long I stayed out on the curb with my plastic bag, I don't remember coming back in the house, all I remember is that feeling of not being good enough. It is this feeling that I hate because I've carried it with me even into adulthood. The times when I let my doubt consume me, the times that I let myself get in my head about not being good enough or pretty enough or smart enough or strong enough—I know it's all rooted in these childhood experiences, and this was just one of many. Knowing now that my mother suffered from mental illness and knowing that she had troubles rationalizing situations and dealing with stress, I know that she would never have intentionally made me feel the way I did many times. It's knowing this that helps me deal with the memories and try to not let them consume me. But it's not easy and it's a constant struggle that I continue to fight.

The craziness was not always directed at us, the kids; often times it was father who bore the brunt of her illness and manic episodes. The neighbours must have thought we were quite the family—the nights my mother would go running out into the street in her bathrobe, yelling at the top of her lungs, crazy stuff like that. And I am allowed to call it crazy because I lived through it. I am not in any means belittling or mocking the mentally ill, just telling it like it was at the time: crazy.

The depression, the extreme OCD, the manic episodes, they were my childhood and they shaped me into who I am today. These DNA moments that I recall, as much as I hate them, I let them through because I need to recognize them, own them and allow them to help me make sense of why I am the way I am. Mental illness has a terrible stigma attached to it. For those who have never been exposed to it, it's hard to understand people that suffer from it. Having been so intimately exposed to it for many years I have a different understanding of it, and although I may be angry at times for having to be exposed to it, I can't change the things that happened, so my only alternative is to embrace them, learn from them and continue to grow from them.

My mom and dad were also very strict parents. Now, when I say strict, I mean not-even-allowed-to-sleep-over-at friends'-houses strict. Talking to boys was a big no-no. If a boy ever called the house asking for my sister or me, we were in big trouble. I was always so jealous of my friends at school who had "cool" parents. They shopped at the cool stores and were able to do sleepovers and talk to boys. I, on the other hand, shopped at discount stores and was scolded if a boy even looked my way. We (my sister and I) got into a lot of trouble growing up; our parents instilled fear in us, so anytime we strayed from our parents' rules, we knew we were going to get yelled at. I think this must be the reason why I am so intimated by people of authority. I'm the kind of person who gets nervous when crossing the border or speaking to a customs officer even though I have nothing to hide. It's as though I revert back to that child who is afraid to ask her parents to go to her friend's house. Sad, so sad. But, hey, at least I can admit it.

In the little town that my parents had settled in, the town that I grew up in, every year there would be a summer festival called the Bread and Honey Festival. It was really the bee's knees. There was a big parade that took place on the Saturday morning that kicked off the opening of the carnival that was set up for the weekend in one of the local parks. So you can imagine how anxious I would get every year around this time, especially in my later years of elementary school. All of my friends were allowed to go the park by themselves and hang out, but not me. I was forced to go with my mom and dad and hang out with them—so embarrassing! I hated every moment of it and it was yet just another time in my life when I felt not cool enough, not good enough to be with the cool kids.

I know that my parents were just trying to protect me from the big, bad evils of the world, but what they inadvertently ended up doing was forcing me to feel the pressure to "fit in." I started smoking at an early age because it was cool and that's what the cool kids were doing. I drank at house parties because I wanted to fit in; I was always trying to be someone other than who I truly was because I was chasing the feeling of acceptance. For all I know, maybe I would have done these things regardless of my parents' parenting style, but maybe I wouldn't have. All I do know is that if I had the chance to go back in time, knowing what I know now, I would have done things differently. I would not have cared as much about what other people thought and would have been a stronger, more confident girl. I say this because I would hope that if that were the case then I would be a little bit stronger of a woman. I got a late start in life when it came to confidence and self-acceptance; it didn't happen easily or overnight, but it did eventually happen. Post-cancer Lina had to go through hell and back again to get here, but, man, was it ever worth it. I am proud of post-cancer Lina—my accomplishments, my outlook on life and how I don't let obstacles get in the way of doing the things I want to do. I am so happy that it is post-cancer Lina that is raising my daughter and I can only hope and pray that I do her justice as a mother. That I never make her feel the way I sometimes felt as a child, that I provide her with the tools and emotional support to become a strong, confident and independent woman. That her growing up will be a different kind of crazy than mine was.

Although my childhood is a little fuzzy at times and I unfortunately recall more of the not-so pleasant moments than the happy ones, I know they did exist; I do have some wonderful memories of my parents in the later years. One moment that I remember very vividly was my first day of radiation treatment. I had already gone through one cycle of chemo. My chemo schedule was one week on, three weeks off. The radiation started during my second month of chemo. Because the radiation was at a hospital in downtown Toronto, that month I had my chemo treatment at the same hospital, which was a different hospital than the one where my surgery and other chemo treatments were done. I remember it being a very long day of waiting. After a long wait time for my radiation session, I had to head over to the chemo floor and wait for my turn there. I had been warned that the chemo would feel different this time around because of the effects of the radiation having been done on the same day. Collectively, the two together were most likely going to make me sicker than each would on its own. Even with the warning I did not expect to become as sick as I did. As soon as they started the chemo injection it was instantaneous sickness. I remember so clearly my dad holding my hand, my mom holding my barf bucket and me crying. I was crying for so many reasons. Crying because I was scared for my life, crying because I was in so much pain and crying because, in the strangest of places, I was bonding with my mom and dad. We were never the kind of family to say the words out loud to one another, but in that moment, I knew that they were saying they loved me and I know if they could, they would have taken my spot in a heartbeat.

My father passed away in December of 2006 after a long four months of suffering in the hospital with ischemic bowel disease. It was very difficult to see my father suffer and deteriorate in front of my eyes. Years after he had held my hand many times when I was sick, it was now time for me to hold his hand while he was sick. One of my DNA moments I have involving my father was a conversation that we had together one day in our backyard. My father was an avid gardener; he would spend countless hours in the yard doing anything and everything. We had a vegetable garden that was probably bigger than most urban lots— he planted everything from potatoes to corn, tomatoes and peppers. We also had berry bushes lining the perimeter of our yard, along with a strawberry patch enclosed by a grape vines. My father was also a master pruner; he could prune trees like nobody's business and would often be called to help out at his friends' homes to prune their trees. All this to say that my father loved being outside, he loved being one with the earth. And since he spent most of his days, weather-permitting, outside, it was also the time that I could chat to him about stuff. I can't recall exactly why we got on the topic of friends this day or exactly how old I was at the time, but I think I must have been in my late teens because it was definitely pre-cancer Lina having this conversation. I remember sitting on the edge of our very large garden bed, the weather was nice out and my father was hunched over, picking green beans off their stems (oh, the green beans—they were so delicious), and he said to me, "Lina, it's better to have as many friends as you can count on one hand than it is to have many." He was such a wise man. He was trying to tell me was that I was better off having a few close friends than a bunch of acquaintances where the friendships were shallow. Such great advice this was; I'm not sure if I fully comprehended the depth of the advice at the time, but reflecting on it now, at an older age, it makes so much sense. I am better off having a handful of true friends, friends who have my back, who love me for who I am and not someone I'm trying to be, than bunch of shallow relationships. Growing up, I struggled a lot with popularity and tried so hard to fit in with everyone, with all the cool kids at school. Unfortunately for me, I lost out on having close friendships with people because I was overly focused on trying to be liked by too many or not the right people. I wish I could remember the context of our conversation that day; for whatever reason my psyche is not allowing me to recall all the details, but at least I recall this advice from my father, advice that has helped me navigate my friendships in my adult life.

Well-known motivational speaker and business philosopher Jim Rohn has spoken and written about how we are the average of the five people we spend the most time with. His statement relates back to the law of averages, which is that the result of any situation will be the average of all outcomes. Post-cancer Lina knows that life is too short to be wasted on getting the approvals of all the people in my life, of trying too hard to maintain a friendship that is not worthy of my time. When I look at my life now, my husband being one of the five people I spend the most time with, the remaining four are friends that I respect, that respect me, that challenge me and push me to be a better me, that love me for who I am, not for what they expect me to be. The five people that I spend the most time with are my closest friends, the number of fingers on one hand. I am surrounding myself now with people who will empower me, not disenfranchise me.

I don't have many regrets in life, but the one regret I do have is that my father never met my little girl. It's not actually a regret because I could not prevent it from happening, but it's a sadness that I will always carry. I was my dad's little girl and I know Liana would have been his little girl, too. Yes, there were many ups and downs growing up, but overall, there was more good than bad, there was food on the table, a safe roof over my head. A "crazy" family we were, but a family that I would not trade in for the world.

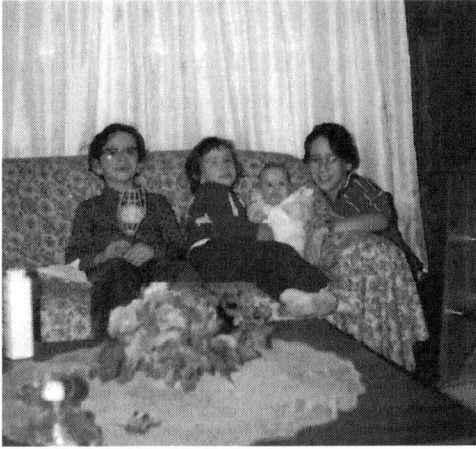

My siblings and I as kids. My sister Nel to the left
of me (the baby) my eldest broth Robert to my
right and my older brother Rick on the far left.

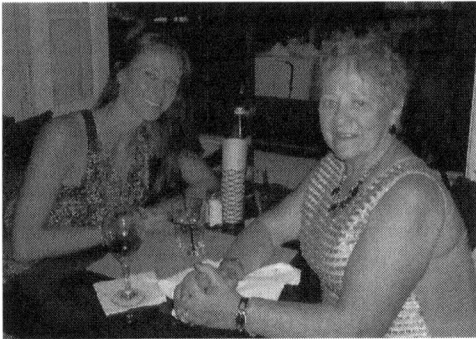

Me and my mom celebrating her 70th
birthday in South Beach Miami.

5 Get Your Ass out of Bed

My sister Nel (Nelia) and I were really close growing up. We did everything together; we shared a bedroom, the same neighbourhood friends and got into the same kinds of trouble. Although there are four years separating us—her being the older one—it never really felt like it. We really were partners in crime as kids. Growing up, there were always four of us who hung out together: my sister who was the oldest, our friend Denise who was a year younger than my sister, Beth who was also a year younger than my sister and then there was me, the youngest of the gang. Denise was our parents' best friends' youngest daughter, so it was only natural that we would be friends, too.

I'm not sure if it was a Portuguese thing, but every Sunday night after dinner, my parents would either host a "*visita*" or go visit someone else—a cousin or a close friend—at their home. At these *visitas*, the adults would wear their Sunday best, oftentimes the clothes that they went to church in earlier that day. They would gather in the kitchen or, on special occasions, the living room (which usually had plastic on all of the furniture) and chat to one another about their village back home and reminisce about old times. A spread of desserts would be displayed for all to enjoy and, depending on the host, coffee and tea or port and whiskey would make its way out for libation. I'm actually laughing out loud as I write this because I'm just realizing now just how nutty this ritual was. I must have never brought this up at school to my English friends or I would have remembered them making fun of my family for doing these *visitas*. Okay, enough laughing at myself, moving on…at these *visitas,* the children would always come along and go play somewhere else in the house. It was really fun to go over Denise's house because her old house, the one that she lived in until the age of about 10 or 11, had the coolest crawl space. It was just off the laundry room in her basement; we could crawl in there and sit for hours talking about our strict parents, our boy crushes, and wondering what life would be like when we were 30. Beth, who lived just a few streets down, would often join us for our Sunday *visitas* and hang out with us, too. Funny how, back then, at the ages of nine, 12 and 13, we would dream about what being 30 would be like. I remember thinking it seemed soooo far away. Would we get married (that is if we would ever be allowed to speak to boys)? What would we be (professionally)? Would we have kids of our own (which we all promised we would allow to talk to boys if they were girls)? Beth was the cool one in the group: she was allowed to talk to boys and have them over. She was allowed out even after the street lights came on and her parents let her have sleepovers! Once we were a bit older, we no longer had to go with my parents to their *visitas*, we were old enough to stay at home and do our own thing. For my sister and me, this was great, because we knew for sure that my parents would be gone for at least two to three hours on Sunday nights, which meant we could go and hang out at Beth's house and, of course, Denise would be there, too.

One summer break, Beth had introduced us to the neighbourhood boys, two brothers who lived down the street from her. In our eyes, they were the coolest guys ever—they wore their Doc Martens and Union Jack shirts with swagger. I can safely say my first crush was to the younger of the two brothers, and sadly everyone in the group knew it. I would be teased about my crush often by the girls, but it didn't bug me, it just fuelled my crush even more. This group of six was pretty tight for many years—even as the older ones went off to high school and got their driver's licences, we would still hang out in each other's basements (correction: Beth's or the boys' basements) and listen to Guns N' Roses and Pearl Jam and smoke cigarettes that were stolen from their parents. The six of us all ended up at different high schools and inevitably, we grew apart, and the tight little clan of six was no longer as it used to be. Because my sister and I ended up going to different high schools, we grew apart slightly, as well—not in a bad way, just in the normal sense of growing up. The four years that separated us became more apparent as we got older; the difference between 15 and 19 was much different than it was at eight and 12. Although we may not have been as close as teens and young adults as we were when we were younger, we were still very connected and relied on each other for advice or to lend an ear when needed.

I would be lying if I told you that I knew how my illness affected her. I never asked her how she was doing with it all and she never really asked me how I was doing with it all. I think the two of us felt scared to bring it up, to show our true emotions. From my perspective, I never shared with anyone how scared I was most of the time. If you recall, I told you in an earlier chapter that when I was released from the hospital and came home, I spent a couple of weeks sleeping with my sister in her bed. Everyone thought it was because I was very weak and needed help in the middle of the night to get up or roll over, but the truth was I was afraid to be alone at night. Thinking back now, I don't know why I never felt like I could talk to her about what I was feeling; if anything, you would think that she would be the one person that I would have felt comfortable doing so with. It probably had a lot more to do with actually voicing my thoughts out loud vs. whom I was going to say them to. If I admitted how I felt, then perhaps I was affirming my truth or my future. Needless to say, although the words may not have been spoken, the silence was understood. I knew that Nel was there to support me even if we did not talk about what was going on.

The day after I woke up from my surgery, my sister had come by the hospital to visit and brought with her matching kerchiefs. At the time, we had no idea if the chemo would cause me to lose my hair or not, so I wore a kerchief to get myself used to the look, just in case I was going to go bald. Knowing that she brought two, one for her and one for me, showed that we were in it together—that I did know.

As life would have it, though, the weeks passed and the weeks turned into months and everyone around me went back to living their regular lives. It became the norm that I would be lying on the couch all day sleeping and resting, shedding weight by the day due to the treatments. The shock and the scare of my situation were no longer as bold as they were in earlier days. Time had gone by, and with time, the normalcy of the situation set in. That, for me, was probably one of the hardest things to go through: watching everyone around me continue on with their lives as I continued to fight. The toughest month for me was month two. During my second month of chemo, my radiation started. Radiation treatment was 25 consecutive days and with each day the treatment would get progressively harder on my body, as the treatment is accumulative. I was warned that by the last week of my radiation I might have to be hospitalized to help support my hydration and feeding via a tube. They warned me that my stomach and esophagus would feel burnt, a raw sensation that would most likely not allow me to swallow fluids or food easily. It was this month that I really took a beating, they were right, with every day, I felt like I was taking a step backwards, every day I was a little weaker and in a little more pain than the day before. There was only one time in my whole cancer experience that I was at peace with death, and it was the last week of month two.

If you have ever read any books about death and dying, you've read that research shows that most people who know they are approaching death are at ease with it. There is a sense of calmness that the dying experience before their passing. I hate to admit it, but I think I went through this myself. During the last week of month two, I was pretty much bedridden, the couch downstairs was too far of a trek, so I stayed in bed. The only getting out of bed was to go to the hospital for my treatment. What they warned me about happening happened; I could not drink or eat, swallowing my own saliva was painful, but I did not want to go the hospital again. That was the last place I wanted to be. I remember lying in bed and feeling this peace that I have since read about—I was at peace with dying. As much as death had scared me initially, being in this state of pain and weakness had opened my mind to the possible inevitable and I was okay with it. Looking back, maybe I was just being weak and giving up the fight; whatever it was, I was okay with it.

It was month three, when now I had no reason to get out of bed because the treatments were over and I had three-weeks off until my next chemo session. My sister had come home from work one day, and I heard her asking my parents where I was. It was dark outside, my bedroom was dark, and she opened my bedroom door, turned on the lights, pulled the covers from over me and yelled, "Get your ass out of bed!" I could hear the bath water running; she was going to force me into the bathtub to take a bath. I don't remember her exact words, but they were something to the effect of "You smell" and "You're giving up." "Get your ass out of bed."

I'm not sure if my sister remembers this moment, but for me it's one of my DNA moments. It was a turning point for me: my support was there. Even though everyone around me including my sister had moved on with their day-to-day lives, they were still there to support me and to help me get through this.

I took that bath that night and woke up the next morning and made my way downstairs to the couch—I was not going to give up, I was going to keep fighting. Who knows how if I would have found the strength to keep going if it was not for that bath that night. Lucky for me, the bath did happen and it was my sister that I have to thank for it.

Even though we were not as close as we were when we were younger, it affirmed to me that my partner in crime had my back. Even though it was not every day that we chatted or hung out, I knew that she was there to kick me in the butt when I needed it and get me back on track.

Thinking back to this moment is a great reminder of how we sometimes drift away from friends or family that we were once very close to, but that, in times of despair, times of hardship, those friends and family members will be there to help you. Even now, much later in our adult lives, Nel and I are nowhere as close as we used to be, and that is okay. That is what I call life. We work, we have families and our days and weeks fill up quickly. But that's not to say that if and when we need each other, we won't be there for each other.

The significance of this bathtub moment holds a heavy weight: it was a time when I had hit rock bottom, a time that I was ready to give up and accept whatever fate was waiting for me, but instead I was forced to snap out of it, to get the fuck up and keep fighting, to wash away my pain and my self-pity and move on. I'm sure you have all had your own type of "bathtub" moment in your life. I've had many since this original one. Times when life has thrown some pretty hard curveballs at me and left me thinking, what now? How do I go on? Or do I just give in? Then it happens: we have that catalyst moment when we snap out of our inner negativity and find a way to move on. The catalyst, the bathtub, whatever it is, it's there. We just need to find it or be pushed into it from a friend or loved one and accept it.

So what do we do with these relationships that have fallen astray? It's often much easier to just push blame on others. We are all guilty of it—blaming the other person for not calling as often as they used to, not emailing as much— but it goes both ways, doesn't it? If you are thinking that, is the other person not thinking it, as well? Maybe, maybe not. The point that I am trying to make is that although relationships go astray sometimes, the history that acts as the foundation to that relationship does not deteriorate—it remains strong and sturdy, so while the structure may not be all that stable, the foundation is solid. Have patience with your relationships; be open to understanding the other person's situation or what they may be going through. And most important, don't lose faith that you can get back to where you once were (if you want it to be). It may just be a little bit different than what it was before.

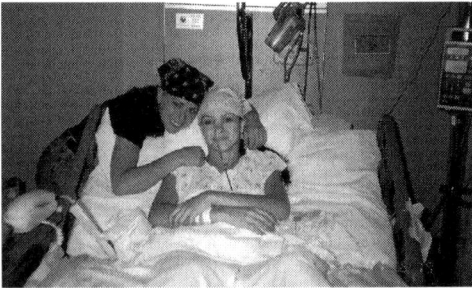

My sister and I wearing our kerchiefs after my surgery.

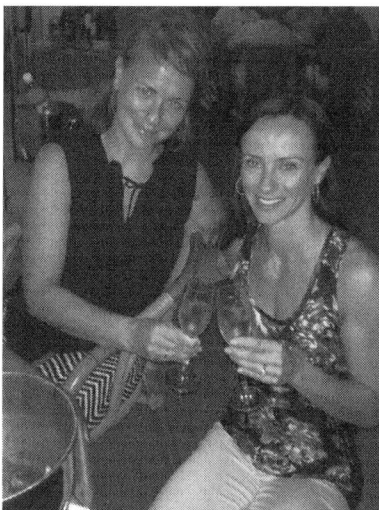

Celebrating my sister's 40th in Cuba

6 Dragons on Water

*"It's a vigorous search for life and well-being
and we embrace the challenge."*
—Gilda's Dragons

Pre-cancer Lina's idea of running shoes was not to go running in them, and rather using them as an accessory for a casual outfit. The only gym that I was familiar with prior to cancer was the one in the community centre where I worked selling memberships; selling memberships was my forte, not actively using one. Post-cancer Lina, though, had a new outlook on life: after having gone through months of utter exhaustion, not having the strength to get out of bed and feeling weaker than an aunt under a horse's hoof, I was determined to never let myself get to that place again. Going through chemo and radiation truly was the best thing that could have happened to me. I wholeheartedly believe that if I had not had that experience, had not felt what I felt, I would not have had my "eureka moment," my transformation from pre- to post-cancer Lina. I was motivated to become a better person, to treat my body like the masterpiece that it should be, to ensure that it was the strongest and most well-equipped piece of machinery that it could ever be so that (fingers and toes crossed) it wouldn't have to endure what it had just gone through again. The new me was not going to let this second chance at life be swept away or taken for granted. By no means do I think that I got cancer because I was inactive or did not go to the gym or take part in some sport, but I do believe that perhaps my recovery and treatments may have been less difficult if I had started off in tip-top shape. Soldiers going into battle are typically at the peak of their performance; they have trained to endure physical and mental toughness and are prepared to cope. Moving forward, I wanted to be a soldier of life, be at my best to allow myself to be my best when it came to enduring life's challenges, big or small. I knew that I had to start doing something, but where to begin? That was the question. I assumed that a team sport would probably be the best place to start; if there were others to rely on and who were relying on me to show up then I would be more inclined to show up. I didn't fully doubt myself but was being realistic that I might need some help to get the ball rolling.

Having no idea where to start, I turned to the web. After searching countless recreational leagues that I could join, I came across a website for dragon boating in Toronto. As with most people, I had no idea what the sport entailed so I did some further research and learned that it was essentially a water sport with 22 people in a large canoe-like boat, 10 on each side, a drummer and a coxswain all working together to propel the boat together as a team for various distance racing. It sounded cool, sounded super fun, so I thought, why not? After some more digging around, I learned that there was a whole society of these dragon boaters residing in Toronto, various teams all paddling out of the waterfront canoe and rowing clubs. Who'd a thunk it? (Keep in mind, this was circa 2003, when the sport was not as popular as it is today.) In my quest to learn more about this sport that for some reason or another had my curiosity piqued, I came across a page that was dedicated to cancer survivors and the sport of dragon boating. All of the teams were comprised of breast cancer survivors. What was the link between breast cancer and dragon boating, I wondered? As it turns out, in 1996 there was a revolution in the way women with breast cancer were treated post-surgery. Prior to 1996, most women were told to avoid strenuous upper body exercise as to avoid lymphedema, a chronic and sometimes painful buildup of fluid under the skin of the arm or shoulder. It was actually a Canadian doctor (props to my fellow Canadian), in BC who set out to prove that exercise could be of benefit to female survivors and started a dragon boat team called *Abreast in a Boat.* Don McKenzie, MD, PhD, a sports medicine physician and exercise physiologist at University of British Columbia was at the forefront of changing the way many breast cancer survivors would live their lives post-surgery. This was all fascinating and super cool, but truthfully I remember thinking, "Great for the breast cancer survivors, but what about me? Why can't I play with them?" Turns out with a few more engine searches I could.

I found that one of the dragon boat racing sites was seeking new paddlers, survivors of any form of cancer to join Gilda's Dragons. Very excited about my find, I quickly called the number and spoke to the team captain and expressed my enthusiasm in joining. I spoke to a wonderful lady who told me all about Gilda's Dragons, a team of female survivors of all types of cancer and of all ages, some of them even two-time survivors! The team is named after Gilda Radner, the American comedian and actor who herself passed away after a battle with ovarian cancer. The team practised on the Toronto waterfront twice a week for one hour and would participate in three to four races per season. I was invited to come out and try a practice. I was so excited! At the time I was still living at home with my parents in Mississauga, a suburb about 30 minutes west of Toronto. I remember my dad once saying that I was crazy for driving so far just to go do a practice where I would probably end up hurting myself. It was typical of my parents to not understand why I wanted to do certain things, especially when it came to fitness or sports. My family was not an athletic one; my parents didn't do anything physical except take the occasional Sunday evening stroll around the block, and my older sister and brothers were never on any sports teams, either. I was not surprised that Dad made the comments that he did; they were not necessarily discouraging, but they sure were not motivating. That being said, I didn't let his lack of support stop me—I didn't care about the drive or the gas money. I was on my way to joining something that, while I didn't know at the time, would turn my life around. Not just in the terms of someone who discovered a new love for fitness and leading a healthy lifestyle, but someone who was willing to try new things and step outside of her comfort zone.

I showed up to my very first practice and remember being so nervous; it was not like me at all to go somewhere on my own where I didn't know anyone, let alone to go do something that I was completely unfamiliar with. This in and of itself was a big deal for me and was an offshoot of my new attitude of, "How bad can it be?" Can't be worse than cancer.

I showed up and looked around for a group of ladies wearing shirts saying "Gilda's Dragons"—and there they were, quite the motley crew of women, ranging in age from the early thirties to, I'm not kidding you, the seventies, in all different shapes and sizes. But they were all so welcoming that my nerves were quickly swept away and replaced with excitement.

I loved our practices out on the water, the beautiful city skyline in the distance, the warmth of the sun on our faces, the energy of 20 women, all whom had once fought for their lives, paddling together and propelling this long boat forward together. Something magical happened every time we stepped into that boat: we were transported to some alternate place where the stresses of the world, the troubles from our days were shielded by our collective strength. Just thinking about it takes me to a happy place and I get goosebumps. We truly were a great group of women with a zest for life that was contagious. There was one woman in particular who had been on the team for two years before me and stayed on for about two years after I joined, who was battling cancer for the second time. Her first battle was with breast cancer, her second with ovarian. This lady was so strong-willed that she actually asked her doctors to speed up her treatments so that she could recover in time to be back on the water for the following year's practices. Seriously—who does that? At the time I thought she was nuts. Now, I realize that she was a passionate gal who knew what made her tick—for her, it was dragon boating, and she would do anything she could to ensure that she was able to continue doing it.

We all have a lesson to learn from her; actually, there are a few lessons we can learn. The first lesson is to suck it up. This poor lady not only had to fight cancer once, but twice. Never once did she complain or play the "poor me" card. She put on her big-girl panties and sucked it up. I truly believe that attitude can help drive our outcomes in life. I believe that if we choose to think positively then our body will remain in a state of positivity which can help it heal. Our brains are so powerful; they drive our every move and decision, so we must remain in a state of positivity, because once an ounce of negativity sneaks its way into your brain, it can set things in motion in a negative direction.

The second lesson is to find something you love to do and do it. Find what makes you tick. Whether it's work or play, life is too short to be doing things that you don't like to do. Okay, I'm going to address those of you who may have just rolled your eyes and thought to yourself, "But I need to put food on the table and support my family—I have to work even though I don't like my job." Yes, that may be true in some circumstances, some of you may not be able to change your job or career and may not love what you do for work, but that does not and should not stop you from taking part in other things that you do love. In fact, I believe that it's especially important for those who are in this situation to find something else that you love to do in your spare time so that you can enjoy life and add balance to your days. If you have to be miserable at work (which I don't recommend at all), then at least find what you are passionate about outside of work. Everyone needs something that challenges them and makes them feel alive. Finding this will help you get through the hours of the day that may not be so enjoyable. For this lady, it was dragon boating that gave her that feeling of being high on life. For some it might not even be a physical activity, it might be painting or bird watching. You may not even know that it's missing right now, but, man, when you find it, you'll wonder how you ever lived without it.

Gilda's Dragons became a second family to me. I spent seven years paddling with them, summers on the lake, winters in a pool. We laughed many times and we cried a few. Unfortunately, we were not immune to tragedy and we lost one of our dragons much too soon. She had an angelic smile and a look in her eyes that was calming. She had battled cancer in her early thirties, was in remission for a few years and succumbed to her second battle before she turned 40. She was a wonderful spirit whom I was privileged to know and paddle with. At her memorial service, everyone who spoke about her mentioned her incredible beauty, both inner and outer. They spoke about her kindness and her willingness to always help others. She wanted us to celebrate her life, not mourn her death. I didn't get to see her in her last weeks, but the team members who did said that she was in good spirits to the end. Her strength and positivity will never be forgotten, and to her and all the others who have lost their battle with pride and dignity, with passion and courage, I dedicate this chapter to you. May you rest in eternal peace doing what you love.

7 H.U.A.

Heard, Understood, Acknowledged. Prior to the fall of 2007, these three words had next to no significance in my life; now, these three words are the very reason why I believe that everyone at some point in their lives should participate in some form of exercise that forces you outside of your comfort zone.

One of the biggest differences between pre- and post-cancer Lina is my passion for fitness and living and promoting a healthy, well-balanced lifestyle—and while I had found fitness years before, my love for fitness was ignited with this boot camp and it all started with what I thought would be just one crazy morning of rolling around in the dirt.

My girlfriend Mandy, who at the time was also my weekend hot yoga buddy, had told me about some boot camp that she had signed up for through a referral from a girl that she had met in a couples' soccer league. Mandy, being the great salesperson that she is, convinced me to come out to "Buddy Day," a free trial session of the boot camp. All I had to do was wake up at 4:45 a.m. to drive 25 minutes to a different city and be prepared to work out and get dirty. Me, being me, not knowing how to say no, said yes. "What's one day of waking up early?" I asked myself. The very next day, I went to bed crazy early to ensure that I could actually roll out of bed at the godforsaken time of a quarter to five to go play with my friend. We carpooled the over 25 km to some big park in the next city, whose only lighting source were the scarce stars in the sky. We parked our cars and I very seriously asked Mandy if this was safe: two girls walking through a dark park to an open field to stand facing east and wait nervously for the "corporal" to arrive and perform roll call. As we approached the opening, I noticed another girl standing completely by herself also facing east and looking a little nervous herself. Well, apparently Mandy and I were not the only crazy girls who had a little too much trust in random strangers that claim to get you in the best shape of your life. And, just like out of some crazy movie, who appeared but a very big (fit) and scary-looking man with his camouflage pants tucked into his military boots, stopwatch around his neck and clipboard in hand. "Here, Corporal," answered Mandy and the other girl after he had called them by their last names. Then it was my turn. He stared at me and very sternly asked me, "What is your last name?" Shyly, I answered, "Miranda," and he very quickly responded, "Do we have hearing issues? What is your last name?" Very smartly this time, I answered back, "Miranda" (insert Spanish accent to pronounce it "*Mee*-randa"). Probably not the best way to have introduced myself to the corporal for the first time, as smart remarks and sharp attitudes were very much frowned upon.

Next, we were introduced to our various exercise equipment that consisted of sandbags, rebars (simulating actual weights of machine guns), long heavy metal poles, a telephone pole (yes, you read that correctly), tires (big ones) and weighted backpacks. We didn't use all of these that very first day, nor did I think I would ever see them again, but as fate would have it, I did, for two wonderful years. After my first experience with this military-style boot camp, I was hooked; as my husband often says, "I drank the Kool-Aid." There was something about that first day that I experienced, some great liberation that I felt being pushed to my limits, being forced out of my comfort zone, and always being told that I could do any exercise and instructed to never to say never. That very night, I signed myself up for the boot camp and for the next two years of my life I woke up before the crack of dawn, rain or shine, hot or cold, and rolled out of bed to be pushed to the limits, to be told that I could do anything that I allowed myself to do.

Boot camp had magically found a way to ignite this spark in me that fuelled a passion for living that I had uncovered after being sick. I became a different person, not just because of the obvious fitness benefits, but because of the mental strength that I had grown. The boot camp had a mission statement: Mission, Team, Self. "Mission" stood for the "missions" that we would perform in our daily exercise activities, "Team" for the platoon of people that worked together to achieve our missions, and lastly, "Self" is self-explanatory. The mindset of camaraderie was engrained in us; we never left any soldier (person) behind. If we had 200 burpees and 300 chin-ups to perform collectively as a platoon, we performed them as a team so that we could achieve our goal. If someone could not run as fast as the others, we always circled back to ensure they weren't left behind. Most important, the boot camp taught me that no matter how hard the mission sounded, I knew that if we worked as a team, we would get it done.

The boot camp was structured that each day of the week would consist of various workouts and, once a week, usually on Friday, we had a Mission Day—the day of the week that I most looked forward to. On Mission Days we would huddle around the corporal and he would lay a map down on the ground, shine his headlamp on it and review our mission of the day. This debrief usually involved a brief description of our scenario, what the mission was, how long we had to complete the mission and who would be in charge of leading the mission. I have to admit I always got a little anxious on Mission Days when my name was called to be the leader. The corporal spoke so fast and moved his fingers around the topographic map so quickly that I was always afraid of missing part of his instructions and potentially causing my platoon to do more exercises than needed—and God forbid if we didn't understand everything the first time around, because if the corporal had to repeat anything he did so as long as we were holding a plank or performing a wall (tree) squat or doing some other sort of stationary hold. Of the many, many missions that we performed, there is one in particular that stands out—a DNA moment, perhaps. It was the dead of winter—a solid 10 to 15 degrees below zero, we were standing around a map in the pitch dark with our headlights on, and my name was called to be the mission lead. On that particular day I remember feeling a little under the weather, a little sluggish and just not fully into being there, and, of course, that was the day that I was picked to be mission lead. The mission involved a 10 kilometre run, hills, trails, sandbags and lots of sit-ups, chin-ups and burpees, all with the end goal of detonating pretend IEDs (improvised explosive devices). The most difficult part of this mission for me was that I would have to ensure that I returned the entire platoon back to the finish point by a designated time; otherwise, we faced consequences for the platoon, and of course being a fitness boot camp, these consequences came in the form of more exercises. I distinctly remember thinking to myself, "How the heck am I going to pull this off?" I could barely make out the route on the map, and I had to organize my platoon according to their running capabilities and ensure that we all completed all of the checkpoint exercises in time. But in the exact same thought, I also recall thinking to myself that I had no choice—there was no time to even think about not doing it because I had to find the strength and energy and capacity to get through it. Moreover, I was not alone. I had my platoon to ensure that it would get done. The reason this particular mission stays so vivid in my memory is because I remember feeling like there was no way that I could get through the next hour and a half of my life, almost like it was impossible, but at the very same time I knew that I would get through it because there was no other option than to get it done. It was this attitude of positivity that was constantly enforced in us every morning which helped me grow into this person that I occasionally have to pinch because I can't believe I actually do all of the things I do.

Our boot camp had a creed that we often recited. One line of the creed that will forever be engrained in my mind and one that I hope will touch you as deeply as it touched me was, "For those who challenge themselves, life has a flavour that the unwilling will never know." Now do me a favour and read it again. Okay, maybe just one more time to make sure that you really absorb the essence of the words. My mission for you is to chase the rainbows in your life. Find those flavours that ultimately only you can find. My catalyst to learning how to push myself beyond my limits and to welcoming the fear of uncertainty and the simultaneous conviction of success was fitness boot camp. Catalysts may not always present themselves so easily in life; you may have to go searching for them. Know that some of them may not be as strong as you hoped and know that some of them may be more than you ever imagined. The key here is to be open to the possibilities and the experiences.

I remember when a new member joined our platoon; he joined in the month of February, which in Toronto is a very cold month and often a month full of snow. Our new member was well over 280 pounds, very tall and looked somewhat nervous or perhaps even second-guessing his choice to come out on that bitter cold, dark morning. His first day happened to be Cardio Day, which meant we were going for a long run. About half a kilometre into our run, it began: the vomiting. Our new member was—well, to say the least—very out of shape and a light jog (actually more of a speed walk) was too much for his body and he vomited quite a few times. Actually he vomited a lot. So why has this memory stuck with me? Because it was this new member's determination to keep on pushing himself and keep on running that I admired so much. He had a will to push through and prove to himself that he could do the task at hand no matter how difficult it was. And even though he ended up walking the latter portion of the run, we were there every step of the way to cheer him on and double back to check on him, and when he finished he had the biggest smile on his face. I was so proud of him and the rest of the platoon for cheering him on and helping him get through that difficult first day. The moral of the story is to keep on pushing and never give up, no matter how tough it may be in the moment, because the feeling of accomplishment when you are done is priceless.

Not only did the boot camp provide me with a new-found flavour of life, it also gave me some great friends, friends that I still have today and cherish in my life. I sometimes think about what my life would be like if I had never said yes to Mandy, if I had never experienced the boot camp. Would I still have found my new flavour of life? Would I have crossed paths with my friends through some alternate avenue? Fortunately, life does not work that way and the "What if?" game only lasts a few seconds before we come back to reality and realize that we are in the moment because it did happen. Retrospective reflection allows us to look at our experiences and learn from them. We can choose to take the good, the bad or the ugly from any experience and dwell, learn or grow from it; the key thing is that without experiences, we wouldn't have the opportunity to do any of (these) things.

My new flavour of life was deeply rooted in the experiences I gained from this boot camp. The camaraderie of the team, the never-quit, never-fail mentality that was ingrained into us every single morning fuelled me and provided the nourishment for my newly developing self: one of growing confidence and security. When the boot camp ended, I was truly saddened, and while I did continue on my fitness journey, I always missed that feeling I had when I finished a session at boot camp—that is, until I found CrossFit.

A couple of years ago, I had been feeling a little disenfranchised with my fitness routine, so I wanted to try something new. I had heard a lot about CrossFit and wanted to see for myself what all the hype was about, and I'm so glad that I did. CrossFit has not only filled that void that I had been feeling with my fitness routines, but it has become part of my family, literally and figuratively. My husband now also CrossFits and our little Liana comes with us every Sunday morning to cheer on her mommy and daddy; she knows that every Sunday we CrossFit. We love the small group setting of our sessions and the vast array of individuals who partake in the sport—young, old, new and elite—are encouraging and encouraged.

I think for me, personally, why I love it so much is similar to my reason for loving the boot camp: because it physically pushes me beyond my comfort level, and forces me to persevere and not quit—it doesn't allow my fear or discomfort to stop me from moving forward. There are so many parallels that can be made between CrossFit and life: the challenges that we are faced with, the sometimes unforeseeable finish, the mental strength that it takes to get through the next step—the skills that I build on in the gym are so transferable in my life.

Life is life, and the truth of the matter is that we often fail at things, but if we don't put ourselves out there and allow for these experiences then we'll never know the outcome. So why not throw yourself out there and experience something different? Maybe it's a boot camp, or maybe it's Number Three on your bucket list—whatever it is, just go for it! The worst that can happen is you find out that you don't like it (but, hey, now you know). Or maybe, just maybe, you'll drink the Kool-Aid and find your new flavour of life.

8 Getting up on Stage

It is definitely common to have stage fright or dislike speaking in front of a crowd. I was no exception. I disliked having to go up in front of people, and I always looked the other way when teachers asked questions because I didn't want my name to be called. I even got sweaty palms as a child and teen having to walk the Eucharist down the aisle at church if my family was selected to do so. Anything that involved large groups of people looking at me would inevitably cause heart palpitations. So, the idea of ever becoming a fitness instructor was nonsense to me. Sure, it was nice to dream about, but to actually think that one day I would get up on stage wearing next to nothing in front of men and women was just a vision of an alternate being in an alternate universe. Well, never say never because it happened!

I can pinpoint the day that I first had the thought of being a fitness instructor. I had joined a GoodLife Fitness® club near my house a few months after I started dragon boating. My endorphins were flowing and I was on a high, feeling great. I joined because I wanted to start doing some more activity outside of my new-found love of sport, and GoodLife Fitness® Clubs in Canada have group exercise programs developed by Les Mills International (LMI) that interested me. There are a variety of classes offered by LMI, some of them being: BODYCOMBAT®, BODYSTEP®, BODYATTACK® and BODYPUMP®. I had tried a few of them but it wasn't until I tried BODYPUMP® that I fell in love. It was similar to meeting someone for the first time and experiencing love at first sight—that feeling of intangible energy that is difficult to put into words. This is what I felt after my first BODYPUMP® class.

BODYPUMP® is a barbell and weights resistance class that works various muscles of the body in blocks of work. The class is broken up into 10 tracks, each with a specific muscular focus and excellently choreographed to energy pumping, feel-good music. I truly will never forget my first class. I stood at the back-left corner to the stage (Does it surprise you that I was at the back?), and, by the time the class was over, I was clapping and thinking to myself, "That will be me one day—I want to be up there providing others with the exact same experience that I just had."

I'd be lying if I said I acted upon this thought of mine anytime soon afterwards. Remember, I was the one who hated being in front of people. I was only a year post-treatment and I was nowhere near the fitness level that I would need to be at to even begin entertaining the idea. That, coupled with the fact that I was still very much consumed with self-doubt meant that the odds of my ever becoming a fitness instructor were actually very low.

Nine years—and a whole lot of experiences later—I found the courage to move forward with my dream: I enrolled in a fitness instructor's course. I am somewhat embarrassed that it took me so long to do this, but in retrospect, I think I needed all of those experiences over the years to mould me into the person that was ready to take the leap. I believe the final tipping point for me was the conclusion of the boot camp that I had been so committed to for the past two years of my life. My confidence had grown by leaps and bounds during my two years with the program that, when it came to an end, I found myself to be somewhat in withdrawal. I was craving to be challenged and to be pushed to new limits. This is when I realized that it was time to finally time to act upon this dream of mine.

I remember it as if it happened yesterday. I was sitting on my couch with my best friend Brittney one evening, enjoying some vino, and I turned to her and said, "What am I waiting for? I should just do it. If I sign up, there will be no turning back. I won't not go to the course because then I'll feel like a total failure." So, I did it, I picked up my laptop and signed up for the course to get my fitness instructors certificate. I finally took the first step to becoming that alternate person that I dreamed about becoming for so long.

It's interesting that I can so vividly recall certain times in my life, when I sometimes can't remember what I ate for breakfast. I'm sure you feel the same way. It's these moments that I make reference to as DNA moments. These are the ones that shape us and help guide us to becoming who we are. They can take us to that fork in the road that forces us to make a decision to go one way or the other. Regardless of what we choose, whether we make the right decision or not, we remember these moments in our lives as being the life-changing ones. Not all DNA moments have to be big and momentous, either. Take this one, for example: it was just me sitting on a couch with my friend, nothing grandiose about it, but I remember it because it was a moment that led to something bigger. It's similar to my first BODYPUMP® class in that, at that moment, I had no idea that I would be storing it away in my bank of memorable DNA moments, but, looking back, it was another one of those experiences that helped push me to become who I am today. I am sure that if you take a minute now and reflect on certain memories from your childhood, your time in post-secondary school or as a young professional, you will automatically have memories pooling into your mind without even trying to recall them. Take one or two of these memories and ask yourself: Did it lead to something bigger? Do you think these memories helped shape you into who you are today? Was it for the better or possibly the worse? What can you do to learn and grow from these experiences?

After having signed up for the course, I was in a bit of a state of disbelief, but I knew it was the right thing to do and the right time in my life to do it. The first day of the course fast approached and I was so nervous driving up to the gym where it was being held. Walking into the studio, I took a deep breath and said to myself, "You can do this." I sat down next to the first person I saw and introduced myself. I quickly learned that she was as nervous as I was. Knowing that it wasn't just me that was filled with doubt provided me with great comfort. I quickly realized after all the introductions that all of us were there for the same reason: a shared love for fitness. We all wanted to be able to provide for others that which we had so happily received from our past and current instructors. Our course instructor was phenomenal; she was a long-time fitness instructor who provided the group with a sense of calmness and empowered us to believe in ourselves. Over the two-week program, we reviewed basic anatomy (which for me wasn't difficult as I have a science background and had taken a few human biology courses in university), but interestingly, what I found the most challenging was the musicality portion of the program. Learning how to listen to music for counts and blocks was new to me and it took some effort for me to train my ears to hear the breaks in music. From there, what was most difficult was learning how to create choreography to match the beats and blocks of music and present it back with pre-beat cueing in mirror-image form. Having to move right but say left was not easy for my brain and body. All in all, the course was really fun and I learned a lot.

Once the course was over, we had one month to review our theory and prepare for a two-hour written exam. Following our written exam, we had to create and teach a one-hour fitness class to a minimum of six participants. We would be graded by our instructor to ensure that we incorporated all of our theory and put it into proper practice. This, for me, was probably one of the most difficult exercises that I have ever had to perform in my life. I know how easy it must sound to you: pick some music, choreograph some moves to the beats, include a warm-up, cardio, strength exercises and cool down—it's not rocket science. But, oh man, I'm telling you, having to do this felt like I was trying to get myself to the moon and back with a pack of batteries and some electrical tape. I had such a difficult time putting my fitness class together, having no dance background and never having been an active participant in aerobic-type fitness classes. I was struggling big time. All in all, it took me just over six weeks to put something together that I had enough confidence to present and be graded on. There were many times that I had thrown my paper and pen at the wall and contemplated giving up, convincing myself that if this was so difficult, then maybe I was just not meant to be doing it. Deep down inside, though, I knew that failure was not an option, so I continued to hammer through my frustrations and pulled myself together to finally book my practical test date and get it over with once and for all.

Standing on the stage for the first time in front of a group of strangers was horrifying. I was so afraid that I was going to forget all of my choreography or totally mess up my moves and be off-beat, but once I hit play and took the first step forward in my warm up, I was on fire. Something turned on inside of me that I had no idea was there; I fell in love with the stage. I felt powerful and in control and loved seeing the sweat drip off the participants' faces.

I had found a new high in life that I had no idea existed.

After my class was finished, my instructor provided me with my score sheet and congratulated me on passing my practical. Having already passed my theoretical exam, it was official: I, Lina Miranda, was a certified fitness instructor. I was now one big step closer to achieving the ultimate dream of becoming a BODYPUMP® instructor.

Now that I was certified, I had to have a game plan on how to become a BODYPUMP® instructor. Through networking and asking lots of questions, I learned that

I essentially had to "audition" with the region's team lead and receive a yay or nay to move forward with training. Luckily, my form and technique were enough to get a yay, so the team lead put my name forward to be added to the list of people for the next phase of BODYPUMP® training. I was so happy for myself; truly, I was on cloud nine to have come so far from being the shy, nervous pre-cancer Lina to being this woman on a mission, this "nothing can stop me" attitude person.

The next BODYPUMP® training that was scheduled for my province was a few months away, which was perfect as it gave me some time to continue to work on my technique and build up my strength so I would be in the best shape possible going into training. I heard from instructors that the training was gruelling and physically taxing, so I wanted to ensure that I could keep up with everyone and not be the weakest link. Before I knew it, the summer had come and gone and it was September. My training was only a few weeks away. The week prior to training, I received my BODYPUMP® package in the mail. It was a DVD with a master class of the release that I would be trained on, along with the CD of music and a booklet with the choreography. I felt so special to have received my first Les Mills package. I was now one of the "elite." The course ran only two days, a full weekend. The first day was a review of technique, musicality and how to properly read the choreography. The second day was focused on cueing and coaching, all sandwiched together with about eight classes in between and a lot of strength training. My group was comprised of a bunch of complete newbies like myself, along with some already trained LMI instructors in other disciplines. It truly was an amazing weekend, learning from the best in the country and sharing the teachings with incredible people. It was an experience that I will certainly hold in my memory bank forever. At the end of the weekend, participants either received a pass or fail. I received my go ahead and was given three months from the end of that weekend to submit a video of myself teaching a full BODYPUMP® class to a group of participants. In order to prepare for the video, our instruction was to shadow other instructors as often as we could and teach as often as we could to gain the experience of teaching, coaching, cueing, and pull it all together in a class that would qualify us for a pass.

I spent about six weeks doing just what was recommended. I shadowed and team taught as much as my body would allow me to in order to gain the experience that I felt was enough for me to tape myself and produce a near-perfect class. I ended up taping myself a total of three times. The first time was a write-off as I made too many mistakes. The addition of a camera filming me added a whole new layer of nerves to my already-nervous state. The second time around was much better but not perfect, so I went for a third and final taping.

One week after my third taping, I ended up in the emergency room with a bout of severe intestinal discomfort. Sadly, I recognized the pain as I had had it before. I was afraid I was experiencing a bowl blockage, which I knew would result in a painful week-long stay in hospital with surgery a possibility.

My instinct was right. The CT scan confirmed that I had a full blockage and would require having a nasogastric (NG) tube put in.

If any of you have ever experienced an NG tube, you know exactly how horrible the experience can be. For those of you who don't know what it is, let me explain: nasogastric intubation is a medical process involving the insertion of a plastic tube through the nose, past the throat, and down into the stomach…and, yes, it is as painful as you are imagining it to be. Once the tube is in place, it's attached to a suction machine that slowly suctions out all the contents of the stomach over a period of days. The goal is to relieve all the pressure from the stomach onto the intestines in the hope that the obstruction/tangling of the bowels will subside. I've been through a lot with respect to medical treatments—heck I've had a baby, too—and I'm telling you, being hooked up to an NG tube for multiple days, seeing the contents of your stomach being pumped out of your nose and stored in this plastic holder is up there on the list of the top horrible experiences to endure in a hospital.

The NG tube was inserted, days went by, CT scans were repeated and unfortunately, my bowels were not cooperating—they were not untangling themselves, as horrible as this was—the one good thing about the situation was that I would be seeing Mr. Handsome again after so many years.

Mr. Handsome was the original surgeon on my case. He was the first one to be notified of my stay in hospital and was ultimately the one who made the final decision that surgery would be needed to rectify my problem. Mr.

Handsome explained that the scar tissue from the original surgery many years ago had narrowed the bowels in some areas and, as such, these narrowed sections were more prone to tangles and obstructions. When NG tubes cannot resolve the issue, surgery is needed to either cut out the parts of the bowel or, if possible, simply untangle the bowels. It was really nice seeing Mr. Handsome after so many years—he still had his calm smile and tender bedside manner. In true Mr. Handsome fashion, he offered to come in on his day off to perform my surgery, even though any of the general surgeons on site were more than capable of handling my case. Knowing that I had to go in for surgery was horrible, but knowing that I'd be in the hands of Mr. Handsome was comforting.

The whole situation really sucked. I had worked so hard over the past year to get to a level of fitness that I was proud of and had allowed me to move forward with fulfilling one of my dreams in life and now, after what felt like a thousand steps forward, I was taking about 10 thousand steps backwards. One week of an NG tube, no solid foods, zero exercise and abdominal surgery was definitely going to set me back. On the bright side, I was in the best shape I could have been in prior to being admitted to the hospital, so I was hoping for a quick recovery.

The surgery went well and I was up and walking the next day. In fact, two days after surgery I was doing stair climbs at the hospital. I'm convinced many people thought I was insane for doing stairs and air squats in the stairwells, but I could care less; I wanted out and I wanted out yesterday. More than ever, this experience really resonated with what I try to preach to others: be the best that you can be in preparation for the unexpected.

All in all, my recovery was not that bad. It did take a couple of months to get my weight and strength back up to where it was before my hospital stay, but I was pleased with my progress. It was probably a good thing that I had something to distract myself with as I was waiting anxiously for my video results. It was really nerve-racking knowing that someone, somewhere was watching my video clip-by-clip, marking my form and every word that came out of my mouth. All the nerves and anticipation were worth it, though, because in early January 2012 I received the email that I had passed my video evaluation and that I was officially a certified BODYPUMP® instructor. It's really hard to put into words how amazing I felt, how proud I was of myself that I had overcome so many obstacles and fears to fulfill a dream of mine that I never thought would happen.

Over the next few months I was given a permanent spot on the schedule at the gym and I had my very own class. I was now the one on stage who had the ability to change lives as much as that one unknowing instructor had changed my life.

Being an LMI certified instructor has its benefits, one of them being what I like to call, "Christmas in August." It's actually a fitness conference that happens once a year in various cities throughout the world where the creators and national instructors from LMI come and host the LMI classes to instructors. Imagine a room with over 1000 instructors, a stage full of excellence and an energy that is unexplainable. That is "Christmas in August." There are very few times that I can recall being so overwhelmed with emotion while working out, and in fact up, until this year, I can only recall two. The first time was after my very first 10K run about two years into my remission, and the other time was after a dragon boat race that we had raced in honour of our dear friend Katherine who had passed. My latest experience was at my first fitness conference—it was track four of the BODYPUMP® class. Track four is the back track, and it is typically done to an upbeat dance type of song and works on moves such as clean and presses, deadlifts and dead rows. It was a mix of the energy in the room, seeing so many people working in unison, hearing the loud euphoric beats consuming my body, and feeling strong and privileged to be doing what I was doing.

And all of it brought me to tears.

No one around me could see my emotion because the room was dark, I was free to let the experience take over and, man, did it feel good. I reflected upon where I was in that moment and where I had been years ago, fighting for my life. My journey, all the ups and downs had led me to that very moment, a moment that consumed with me with a pure and utter appreciation for life.

Fast forward five years, to this past year, I won a competition to be a shadow presenter on stage at this very conference that I just wrote about. I was selected to be up on stage with the best of the best and look out at a sea of hundreds of instructors. If anyone had told me years ago while I was contemplating becoming an instructor that I would one day be up on stage at the conference presenting, I would have thought they had gone mad. To this very point, I am reminded that in life, sometimes the unthinkable can become reality. With enough dedication, will and the openess to put yourself out there, regardless of the potential to fail, good things can happen. Never say never.

Life is what drives us. It motivates us to keep doing things to live outside of our comfort zones, to try new things, to meet new people and create wonderful memories. Life is not always rainbows and Skittles. It's not always easy, but what can help you find the rainbow is your attitude and your openness to find the sweetness that it absolutely holds.

I challenge you to take that leap, live your dream, or at least try so that you know you did all that you could and have no regrets. Along the way, remember to keep training, because life is and will always be your greatest competition.

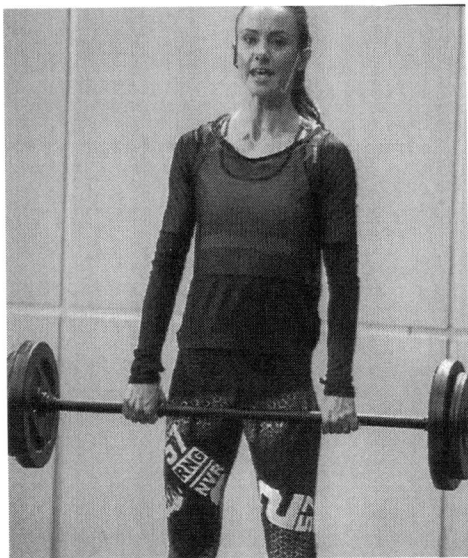

Me teaching a class

9 Oh, Shit

I shit you not; the email below is for real and has not been doctored at all by me for the purpose of this book. One of my best friends, partner is crime, and running partner Brit sent in this email after what was yet another close call in the park. The funny thing about this email is that if you know anything about Toronto's late mayor, you know that Mr. Ford was most likely not a runner and I'd be willing to bet money that he had never been in High Park in need of a bathroom at 6:00 am...then again, maybe he had.

> **Sent:** June 16, 2011 11:14 AM
> **To:** mayor_ford@toronto.ca
> **Cc:** councillor_perks@toronto.ca
> **Subject:** Issue with public washrooms
>
> Dear Mr. Ford:
>
> It is with great frustration I am writing you with regards to the «hours of operation» of public washrooms in Toronto›s parks, particularly High Park, and along the lakeshore. I know I am not the first complaint regarding this matter, so what does it take for

you to reconsider the current procedures in place?

It is no secret that Toronto residents love High Park and the lakeshore for the purpose of exercise. Have you ever been in the park at 6:00 a.m.? You may find it surprising how busy the park is at this time, and how it quickly empties out shortly after 7:00 a.m., just in time for the washrooms to (start to) open up. By the time they finish their rounds, it could be close to 8:00 a.m. before they are all open. I understand issues of safety and maintenance, but there is a solution to every problem, whether it be opening the washrooms an hour earlier, or looking into other methods such as pay toilets (which have been known to work in Europe). My main question to you is, would you prefer human feces throughout the park?

It is unfair to the man at The Grenadier who starts his morning by denying desperate runners to use the washroom before opening. It is unfair to the poor woman I witnessed this morning as she was on the brink of tears in what I assume was hopeless fear of "squatting" in public. It's simple science: exercise makes you go to the bathroom. Again, I know I am not the first complaint on this matter, and I am certain that I will not be the last if something isn't rectified.

I thank you for your serious consideration of this issue and look forward to your response.

Regards,
Brittney

So any of you that run or know people that run know that running can be mother nature's version of a laxative—you know it can get things moving down there. Couple that with the time of day, specifically, first thing in the morning, along with someone who has a compromised digestive system and you get what I call a recipe for the shits. And I'm not talking just a normal number two, an "Oh, I feel it coming on but I have time to finish reading this article in the paper" kind of number two, I'm talking the "Oh my God, it's coming NO…I can't hold it anymore!" kind of number two.

There are pros and cons to every scenario in life; for post-cancer Lina, the pro was my new-found love for fitness and being addicted to the high of endorphins. The con, well, let's just say it was leaving modesty out the door and going to the bathroom in public places far more times than I would like to admit. Running never came easy to me—running around my block a few times for about 20 minutes was pretty much all I could handle when I started out.

I had just broken up with my boyfriend of five years when I met my husband. He was a super cool guy with really nice legs, abs of steel and chiselled cheekbones—turns out this great physique of his came from all of his sports training. Not only was he all-around athletic and excelled at every sport, he was playing semi–pro soccer (pretty much the highest level in Canada you could play while holding a full-time job elsewhere). All of this is to say that I had found the perfect person to help me with my running. During our early courtship, Luch and I decided that we should register for a 10K race. What better race to run than the 10K Canadian Cancer Society race in Toronto. Luch was fantastic and helped me train leading up to the date. The day of the race I was nervous as shit (pardon the association to the topic of this chapter). Running 10K to me would be like running a marathon to someone who had only every run a half; it seemed impossible. But, this was post-cancer Lina we are talking about and post-cancer Lina was up for any challenge. At around the 7K mark, I remember feeling like death—my body was aching everywhere! I wanted it to end; I was convinced that the "runner's high" that all runners talk about was completely made up to brainwash themselves into loving something that was so hard. At the kilometre markers throughout the race, there were lovely volunteers who, God bless their souls, they were just trying to cheer everyone on for this amazing cause. It was there at the 7K mark that a dear old man said to me as I ran by with Luch, "Keep going, dear, you're almost there." What was my response to him? Something that to this day, Luch still brings up at dinner parties: "No, we're fucking not!" Oh yes, I snapped on the poor old man in a way that shocked Luch and probably scarred that dear volunteer. Fast forward 3K and we did cross the finish line, and when I did, it was an instantaneous water fountain of tears. I was so overcome with emotion I could not stop myself. The volunteers were probably thinking that I had twisted my ankle or something, but no, I was just overjoyed with finishing, with being alive and with, yes, running. I'd finally experienced that euphoria that runners talk about: the "runner's high."

So my love for running progressed slowly over the years. I enjoyed my runs as it gave me time to myself to think and to listen to music that would transport me to another place. It was during my time at boot camp that I and another girlfriend and fellow boot camper decided to undertake our first half marathon. We signed up for the Army Run, which takes place in Ottawa to commemorate our country's fallen, wounded and active soldiers. We ran a lot in our boot camp—and I'm not just talking about normal running that normal people do. We ran with weighted rebars, we ran with weighted backpacks, hell, we ran with a telephone pole once. It was on these early morning runs that I learned how to become one with nature. There were a couple of times (I will never admit out loud to anyone exactly how many times) that I would have to run off in another direction to go do my business. I actually got to the point where I was carrying toilet paper with me in my pockets because I knew I would need it. I didn't mind so much having to do my business in the great outdoors during the boot camp runs because it was usually still pitch dark outside and we were usually deep in the dense sections of the park where there were plenty of trees or bushes to hide behind. Unlike the above-mentioned scenario that my dear friend Brit was writing to our late mayor about.

One of my friends, Paul, whom I had met during my boot camp years had run the Mississauga half marathon with Brit and me one year and so the following year, he sent me an email saying, "Lina, I'm going to run my first full marathon—do you and Brit want to cheer me on at the finish line?" Having received this email in enough time to register for the run, I convinced Brit that she and I should run the half, which would give us plenty of time to stretch and have a bite to eat before cheering on Paul at the finish line. Now one would assume that since he did not mention specifically which marathon he was running that he was referring to the same race that we had ran together the year before, right? WRONG. It was not until the week before the race when I offered to pick up his race kit that I realized that he had registered for the Toronto Marathon, and Brit and I were registered for the Mississauga Half Marathon, which were both happening on the same day! We really had no intention of running that half, nor were we even prepared. Neither of us had really been running consistently, let alone long distances; we were really only going to "suck it up" and do the half because we wanted to be there for our friend at the start of the race. That being said, Brit and I ran the half in a pretty decent time: we crossed the finish line in 2:02, which for not really training at all, was pretty darn good.

Both Luch and Paolo, Brit's husband, were at the finish line cheering us on. Paolo, who was a competitive runner in university and worked as a fitness coach for major league soccer, was so impressed by what we could do without any formal long-distance training that he was convinced we could break 1:50 with training, and thus began the start to what soon became a very grueling training period. Paolo took us on as his pet project: Operation Whip These Girls into Running Machines. We had a formal training regime made up for us that consisted of four days of training, sprints, hills, Fartleks, and long runs. Brit and I were waking up early to ensure that we got our training in, especially on days when we knew we would be stuck working late. All this lead-up and explanation to bring me back to the morning of the email. It was hill training day for Brit and me and the perfect hill for training is in High Park—it's about 700 metres with a perfect incline. We would sprint up the hill then run back down multiple times. Well, needless to say, I had all of the elements for the perfect shit brewing. It was early morning, I was training hard, and I have a compromised digestive system—so, yes, it was inevitable that I was going to have to go. It probably was not until the last hill that I remember saying to Brit, "Oh, no…it's happening. I have to go." By that time, the sun had risen and the traffic in the park was picking up with plenty of runners and people walking their dogs. To boot, that hill was smack dab in the middle of the park, no real good hiding place to have to do my business. At the top of the hill there is a crossroads and at the other end of the street is a parking lot for the park café. The café opened at 7:00 a.m. I looked at my watch: it was 6:45. I saw an older gentleman wiping down the chairs on the patio—perfect, I thought! Surely he would let me in to use the bathroom. I walked up to the man, clinching my but cheeks, and very politely asked if I could use the facilities inside, to which he very rudely said no. I, now crossing my legs, told him that I would stay and have breakfast at the café, but in the meantime I really needed to use the facilities. He again, without the slightest hint of humanity, said "NO, we are not open yet." And that's when it happened: the fiery side of me came out and without even thinking I yelled back, "Fine, then I will just have to take a shit on your front lawn!" I walked away like a two-year-old having a temper tantrum, stamping my feet (and clenching my bum). I did not end up squatting on the front lawn of the café; instead, I yelled at Brit to get the car and get the hell out of there because I was minutes away from dropping a bomb. Thankfully, we made it to the gas station down the street.

So where is the connection? Why share my early morning bowel issues with you? For one, the story of my first race houses one of my DNA moments, the one of me crossing the finish line of my first 10K run is a significant one because it reminds me so much of the transformation between pre- and post-cancer Lina. Pre-cancer Lina would have not only told that volunteer where to go, but she would have stopped running and maybe even have walked off the race course. Post-cancer Lina, well, she still swore a lot and was nasty to the volunteer, but she fought through the physical pain and crossed the finish line, crossing to a moment of pure emotion, joy and satisfaction. Often times we face situations in life where it may appear easier to give up than to keep fighting. The instant satisfaction of giving up, being free from what it is that we are fighting through is just that, instant…but short-lived. It's a high that has an almost instantaneous low. On the flip side, the satisfaction that you get from completing something is long-lasting. Its effects will stay with you and provide you with the strength to get through the next difficult situation. Courage, bravery, emotional and mental tough-ness, all similar to physical toughness, require training;

the more you train, the easier it will get and the stronger you will become.

Whether it is training to improve a race time, which I might add, worked; I ran a half marathon later that year and broke 1:50. Or, it is learning a new skill at work, the moral of the story is that you have to put in the time, despite how hard, uncomfortable, or time consuming the training may be. For me, having to embrace my bowel issues in public was not easy and I knew that the chances of me having to "go" much outweighed the chances of me not having to "go", but I stuck with the training because I wanted to reap the rewards. Whatever goal you might have set for yourself, personally or professionally, see past the obstacles and envision the outcome.

10 Where is the Exit Sign?

A DNA moment does not have to be actually lived by you in order to be classified as one. A DNA moment could be someone else's experience that may (or may not) have shaped their lives but when shared with you, for one reason or another becomes a DNA moment. For all you *Star Trek* fans out there, consider it a Vulcan mind meld: "My mind to your mind, my thoughts to your thoughts." Only in the real world, we don't need to be placing our fingers on each other's temples to experience this out of body experience; rather, we can simply talk and share our experiences. Going back to my definition of a DNA moment, it is a moment that intrinsically gets filed away without any conscious support from our psyche. It is a moment that has shaped or will help to shape our future self by affecting the decisions we choose to make. DNA moments are those moments that, without having to think about them, always pop up from our memory banks. They are the moments that we often reflect back on, the ones that we replay over and over again, the specific moments or experiences in our lives that we recall vividly, whether they were good or bad. These are the moments that are shaping the very essence of who we are. Do I believe that DNA moments have a special power to magically transform us into a better version of us? Nope. If that were the case then we would be experiencing a macroevolution of a superior human race. DNA moments are simply there to act as the internal mediator to our decisions. Take, for example, my greatest DNA moment—or should I say moments (plural)—in my life: fighting cancer. If I had to pick one of the many DNA moments from the overall experience, I would have to say it was the day that I was given my odds for survival. I will never, ever forget the moment that I was told I had a one in five chance of a five-year survival. This was the beginning of the morphing of pre-cancer Lina to post-cancer Lina. The moment when pre-cancer Lina, who probably would have given up and crawled under a rock or turned to not-so–appropriate behaviour to cope with her situation, morphed into this strong person who decided that she WOULD beat the odds and she WOULD live past five years. Never wanting to experience that moment again, fast forward a year…Never wanting to go through surgery, chemo and radiation again, post-cancer Lina underwent a dramatic transformation. Looking back, my transformation could have ended up in the polar opposite direction. I could have ended up defeated and angry at the world for what I was going through, given up and conceded to "fate."

This chapter is based on a moment that my husband experienced one day at work. It's a moment that we often, as a couple, will reflect on when making career-based decisions. It happened back when my husband was a senior manager working for a global IT manufacturing company. The year leading up to this moment, he had taken on a special project that was a fantastic opportunity for him in his career: he had been charged with leading a team of internal executives and directors on a special pilot consulting project with another global manufacturing company. Luch's expertise is supply chain optimization; he is a true "out of the box" thinker who can envision things on a macro level but has the expertise to execute at the micro level. At this pont in his career, now filling two roles, I watched my husband slowly drifting away from who I knew him to be. He was tired, overworked and downright miserable at the fact that his work life was overtaking his personal life. It was at this time that I coined a term, "Asiaitis." Definition: *Inflamation of the body caused by travelling to Asia for business way too often, resulting in bad moods, a short temper and pretty much an altered state of self.* Asiaitis would last for about two to three days every time Luch came back from one of his trips to Asia; he did not adapt well to the long flight times and jetlag. During a bout of Asiaitis, I would keep our conversations to a minimum and try my best not to be sarcastic, poke fun or enter into debates with him as I would most likely get my head chewed off and be sent to the dog house for no real reason.

One day Luch was called into his VP's office to have an informal chat about work and career development. The conversation started out fine from what Luch could recall—the VP was talking about the qualities that a good leader should have and the path that one should take in order to continue to grow and climb the corporate ladder. This was fantastic, I remember Luch thinking; he was getting some really good insight from a leader in his company. The VP then shared a story about one night when he came home from work (and for him at the time of this story, coming home meant flying home for the weekend as he was working out of town Monday to Friday on an off-site project) and his wife sat him down to discuss their living arrangement and the direction their marriage was going in. He went on to say that his wife questioned his love for her and their family and asked him to make a decision: to choose between her and his work, because at the rate that they were going she didn't feel that she could maintain the relationship. Luch, being the kind of man he is, one who puts his family above all else and has values that are deeply rooted in respect and loyalty, then almost fell off his chair when his VP said what he said next: "Luch, I told my wife that night that I chose my career and that if she was not okay with being second place, then we should not be together." The VP went on to talk about how men had to make difficult decisions in life and if they wanted their careers to continue to grow then sometimes they would just have to do whatever it took. It was somewhere in the middle of all of this unsolicited advice that Luch remembered thinking to himself, "Where the heck is the exit sign?" and "Please, God, let there be a fire alarm to get me out of this office now!"

When Luch came home that night from the now infamous "Where is the exit sign?" meeting, he was still in shock from all the advice that he had been given. The one thing that he did take away from that meeting—actually, what we both took away from that meeting—was knowing exactly what we never wanted to become. Since then, anytime that Luch or I have had to make a career-based decision, whether it involved changing teams, taking on new projects, or moving companies, we have always reflected back on that moment. If we felt that making the move would steer us in the direction of becoming people like the infamous VP, or put us in an environment that favoured such values and beliefs, then our decision was an easy one to make. As the old saying goes, "Knowing what you don't want is the first step in learning what you do."

And for those of you who are curious to know if Luch still works for that VP and company, the answer is heck, no.

11   Oh, Baby, Baby

Why is it that what comes so easily to some, can be such a challenge for others? Why is it that something you spend most of your early adult years trying to prevent can one day be so hard to make happen? Why is it that two healthy, smart, well-educated and dependable people can have so much trouble conceiving a baby? Was it our fault? Did we wait too long?

No, we were still young—33 and 35 is by no stretch old, not even in fertility years. We may not have been spring chickens, but neither are other couples who seem to sneeze and get pregnant, so the question remains: Why us?

Luch and I made the conscious decision to get married young. We wanted to spend many years together, alone, travelling the world with no responsibilities. We wanted to establish ourselves in our careers and ensure that we were in a good and safe place before bringing little ones into the world. We did just that. We were married in 2005 after a short courtship of one year and two months and an engagement of the same length of time. I was 25 and Luch was 27. We were young to be getting married compared to most of our other friends who were not even in serious relationships, but as the cliché goes, "When you know, you know," so why put off the inevitable? As a young couple our marriage blossomed every year. Our bond only strengthened as the years went by. We enjoyed many wonderful trips to countries around the world and experienced many firsts together, both alone and with good friends. Incredible memories of surfing in Hawaii, zip-lining in Costa Rica and sobering up multiple times in one day as we visited the wineries in Mendoza bring such a sweet smile to my face. The idea of having children was always something we talked about. In fact, if it were up to Luch, I think we would have started trying to get pregnant sooner than we did. I never felt quite ready until I was about 31. Before then, I'd be lying if I said I was completely ready to be a parent. I know that no one ever is completely ready, but I was not fully convinced yet that I wanted to forgo the exciting life that Luch and I were living. Enjoying the past eight years together, doing exactly what we wanted when we wanted, was very appealing to me to continue to keep doing. And, if I'm being completely honest, I was not ready to give up my body. I loved working out and training hard, and I was not ready to give all of that up.

I'm sure right now, I've got half of you reading this book thinking to yourself that I am the biggest, most selfish bitch you've ever read about, one who is so vain and selfish that she would choose exercise and physical appearance over reproduction. The other half of you are probably thinking, finally, someone has had the "*heuvos*" (eggs in Spanish a.k.a "balls") to admit their thoughts out loud and are grateful that they are not alone for feeling the same way.

Shortly after turning 31, I started to have secret conversations with myself and would deliberate on the topic of kids. At the time, my older sister was trying to conceive with her husband and she had very gently reminded me that conceiving does not always go the way you plan, and that if we were thinking of having children, Luch and I should consider trying sooner than later. This struck a chord with me. The thought that it may take us years to conceive was scarier than the thought of conceiving right away. Then it just happened a few months later, I woke up one day and I knew that the time had come that I was ready, ready to share my love and passion for life and for my husband with someone else, someone that we could bring into this world together. My nighttime mental deliberations also brought back some conversations that I had had many years ago while going through my cancer treatments. I recalled being told by my radiologist at Princess Margaret Hospital in Toronto that one day when I was older and in my family planning years, to remember that the radiation I underwent may have scattered to my reproductive areas and that it could cause reproductive problems in the future. Having this in the back of my mind, coupled with the fact that I finally felt emotionally ready to become a parent had my biological clock on full alarm and I was not hitting snooze anymore.

And so the joy of baby making was in full swing. Counting cycles, trying to be in tune with my body—it was all so confusing in the beginning. My friends who already had children would ask me if I ever felt my ovaries. Felt my ovaries? What were they smoking? I was that lucky girl who never had menstrual cramps, never had tender breasts, had no idea when my ovaries were ovulating; I only ever knew when I got my period literally at the moment

I got my period. My body, unlike those of my friends, did not talk to me. This made monitoring my cycle and peak ovulation time a little more difficult. What it did do is make Luch a very happy man. "O time" (ovulation time) was Luch's favourite time of the month for many months. After many months of thinking I was pregnant because I thought my period was late, I began to realize that I had irregularly long menstrual cycles. The average cycle is anywhere from 28 to 35 days; mine were averaging 40 to 55 days. Clearly, I needed help in narrowing down my O time. And what should any intelligent women do when she is having girl issues? Why, she should enlist the advice of the other women in her life, so I did just that. The consensus was to start a basal temperature diary and to invest in ovulation sticks that would tell me when I was ovulating. Well, as luck would have it, my basal temperature when plotted daily over a month's time looked more like the QT interval of a heartbeat than what any sort of normal basal temperature fertility graph should look like. As for the ovulations sticks, to be honest, I felt like I was literally pissing my money away because I never seemed to get a positive reading. But being who I am, persistent and hard-headed, I continued to piss my money away. This brings me to remember a time that we were in Las Vegas celebrating a couple's stag and doe. I was convinced that the time we would be in Vegas was right around my O time, but having forgotten my test strips at home I had to make a special trip to the convenience store in Caesar's Palace. My girlfriend and I stood at the checkout line with a bottle of gin, tonic, potato chips, and a box of ovulation testing sticks. I remember laughing with my girlfriend, saying that the checkout girl must have thought that we were the smartest girls in Vegas—girls who actually tested to make sure they weren't ovulating before going out on a Friday night to hit the clubs. Little did she know it was for the complete opposite reason.

After a year and a half of QT temperature graphs and countless boxes of ovulation test strips, I finally came to the conclusion that Luch and I should probably see what tools we had; not borrow trouble, but simply ensure that at least the tools in our toolbox were sufficiently working. I had my family physician refer me to one of the top fertility clinics in Toronto, a well-known, world-renowned clinic. Our first appointment was in the fall of 2012. I had just turned 33 and loved that everyone kept calling me young at the clinic—it was quite the ego booster. Our visit was actually very educational; I learned something that I am about to share with all of you, that you must all share with any female you know who may have either of the following two things in her reproductive toolbox. First, I learned that some types of chemotherapy may have an effect on female fertility. Why was I never told this by any of my oncology physicians? I always prided myself on being a well-read cancer patient; clearly, I'd skipped the chapter on the effects of chemotherapy on female fertility. I had known about the potential for scatter radiation to have an effect on my fertility, but never thought that the chemo would play a role as well. Turns out that the type of chemo I had is thought to have a low risk of causing infertility. That being said, low risk is still a risk, and I think I should have known this. The second "aha" moment we had at our appointment was learning that onset of menopause is hereditary.

My mother went into early menopause—I remember this fact clearly because she had me at the age of 37 and she remembers a year later, as I was learning to walk, she was already experiencing the first signs of menopause. Two huge risk factors were thrown at Luch and I that we had never considered before, and all of a sudden our toolbox was looking a little sparse.

Numerous tests later, we were relieved to find out that our tools appeared to be in fine working order—insert sigh of relief here. Our doctor had chosen a moderately aggressive treatment path for us. We would first try to normalize my menstrual cycles with hormones and have a few goes at "timed sexual relations," or as Luch liked to call it, "O time," and, if necessary, follow this up with two to three cycles of intrauterine insemination (IUI), which, if necessary, would be followed by in vitro fertilization (IVF). Surely, with the proper working tools, I thought we would never end up at the IVF stage, but of course, as life would have it, we did end up there. My official diagnosis was abdominal scarring impeding necessary movement of the fallopian tubes for egg release. Great! I should have known that my surgeries, surgeries that essentially saved my life, would now impede me from creating a life. Ironic, isn't it?!

After six months of trying less aggressive fertility treatments, we were advised that the only cure to my diagnosis was to go with IVF, to get the eggs out of my movement-impaired fallopian tubes, which meant more poking, more hormones, a crazier rollercoaster ride of emotions. After our first IVF embryo transfer, we were convinced that we were pregnant—if there was nothing else wrong with us, and we had perfect little embryos, why would we not get pregnant? That is a question we'll never have an answer to, but it is definitely an experience that got me questioning whether we would ever be able to conceive and achieve a viable pregnancy. Our first attepmt at IVF failed, we had what they call a chemical pregnancy; it lasted only 2 weeks. I had contemplated taking the summer off from the fertility clinic. I was tired, I was done with the all the clinic visits, the hormones, the "taking it easy" at the gym. I wanted my life back, I wanted to know what it felt like to not be bloated from all the injections. I had forgotten what it was like to not have to worry about taking my meds or not sweating too much during a workout because I may be sweating out the hormones. I forgot what my favourite red wine tasted like. I was done. Emotionally and physically done.

Inertia—when at rest, there is a tendency to stay at rest—it's what I preach to my members at the gym every time we are doing tricep dips or lunges and the muscles are burning and screaming at you to stop, I coach: "Don't stop, keep going, fight through—it will be even harder to get started if you stop." Well, if I was going to preach it, I should sure as heck live it. I decided that I would not take a break and continue right away the following month and try IVF again, lucky number two.

Fast forward four weeks later and we received the phone call from the clinic; it was a very long two weeks of waiting to get our preliminary pregnancy results, but we finally got them. We received the phone call on a late Friday afternoon that my beta levels were 181. Anything over four is considered positive, and anything over 100 is considered to be a strong positive. We were pregnant. We had finally completed our build.

The cool thing about going to a fertility clinic is knowing that you are pregnant so early, earlier than you would ever find out if you weren't at a clinic. Every two days after the initial blood test, I would go back for further testing and we would hope to see the expected doubling of numbers, which we did.

Then I received scare number one. Shortly after my fourth blood test, which was done four days after the third, I received a phone call from the clinic nurse stating that the doctor was concerned with the latest blood results: my HCG levels had not quadrupled in the four days as expected and so they were concerned that I may have an ectopic pregnancy. I was instructed to go in the following Monday morning for my first internal ultrasound so they could do some investigating. I remember trying my best not to stress that weekend at the thought that I may not actually have a viable pregnancy. I had to call upon post-cancer Lina to be strong and not let the weak and worrisome pre-cancer Lina take over my thoughts and emotions. Monday morning could not have come any sooner, and I will never forget bursting into tears when I heard the ultrasound tech say, "Congratulations, I see one little heartbeat." Our little embryo—"Brio," as we nicknamed him/her—had nestled its way perfectly into the right place in my uterus.

A week later, I had a second scare. Luch and I had flown to Calgary for his best friend's wedding. I had purchased not one, but two stunning designer dresses for this wedding— one for the ceremony and one for the reception. They were my first two real designer dresses and I was so excited to wear them. On the Saturday morning of the wedding, I woke up and went to the bathroom. After wiping and looking in the toilet (sorry, TMI), I noticed that I was bleeding. Of course I started to panic, and my mind immediately went to the worst-case scenario—I thought I was miscarrying. We called our doctor back in Toronto right away and he calmed me down, explaining that I should stay positive and that the fact that I had no abdominal or lower back pain was a good sign, but that I should rest and stay in bed for the rest of the weekend, and first thing Monday morning I was to see him at the clinic. Monday morning could not have come soon enough. I found myself just one week after my last anxious visit, lying on an examining table and waiting for another internal ultrasound. "Baby is just fine and heart is beating strong"—the words that I was so praying to hear. How could it be that after only seven weeks of being pregnant I was already so much in love with our little Brio? The relief swept over both of us. The bad news was that I did have a noticeable blood clot in my uterus that resulted in my doctor putting me on bed rest for one week until I went back to see him to have the clot re-assessed.

It was that week that I had to make one of my most difficult decisions. In some women's eyes, my decision may have been a no-brainer; but to me, it was a difficult one. I made the decision to remove myself from the summer schedule of teaching at the gym. The one thing that I loved to do so much, the thing that I did not consider work because it brought me such joy and fulfillment, I chose to stop doing. Teaching my weight exercise classes even with light weights can be very strenuous and demanded a lot of energy from me. It was best that I let my little Brio settle into its new home before I did anything that might disrupt its movement. After 1 week of bed rest and 4 weeks of little to light activity, my blood clot was completely gone and I was cleared to go back to my regular activities.

Fast forward 15 weeks, Luch and I were sitting in a tiny, dark ultrasound room after a few walks around the hospital, a couple of stair climbs and an indulgence of sugary treats. I was lying back down on the table hoping that all of my above-noted efforts were enough to get Brio to open up those legs. The efforts were a success and we were told that we were having a little girl! I instantly started to cry out of joy, love and excitement; my hubby, on the other hand, remained poker-faced, expressionless; in fact, if I remember correctly he went pale. I quickly began to feel the awkwardness in the room build. I remember thinking to myself that this poor technician probably thinks I'm married to some ass of a husband who really wanted a boy and is upset to hear the news that we were having a girl. I quickly got myself dressed as fast as I could so I could get Luch alone and find out what was up with his reaction. We barely made it out the door when he turned to me and said, "Promise me you'll teach her not to be promiscuous and how to be a good girl." Turns out Luch's poker face was more about fear than it was disappointment. The poor guy just realized that he was going to be a daddy to a little girl and was immediately filled with all the trepidations that came with being one.

In our follow-up visit to the OB, we were delighted to hear that all of the testing had come back normal and that our little girl was cooking on schedule with no areas of concern, BUT—and I feel that when it comes to me and my health there is always a "but"—I was told I had placenta previa. Placenta previa is when the placenta is lying low in the uterus and covering the cervix. Most women's placenta tends to move as the uterus gets bigger; only a small percentage actually end up having true placenta previa. Further in the pregnancy, we would do another ultrasound to determine what percentage I fell into. I'll give you one gues…YEP, the results of that later test showed full placenta previa. The placenta had not moved at all; it was completely covering my cervix. All this to say that a vaginal delivery was out of the question for me and I was being booked for a C-section three weeks prior to my due date to prevent me from going into natural labour, which could cause severe and in some cases life threatening haemorrhaging.

I've mentioned this before, but I am somewhat of a religious girl and I do believe that God works in mysterious ways. Week 27 of my pregnancy, God was at work, and he managed to get me to roll my ankle, causing me to snap my fifth metatarsal in half, which resulted in me having to be in a cast for six weeks. I was devastated at the time. My pregnancy had been going so well. I felt awesome, never sick, never tired, was still keeping active and carrying on with most of my activities, and now a cast! It was horrible; wobbling around with crutches and being seven months pregnant was no easy feat. But as I mentioned above, I believe it was God's way of saying, "SLOW DOWN!" My C-section was scheduled for Jan 20, and on January 16, at approximately 5:25 p.m., I had gotten up from my office chair at home to go to the kitchen to get a snack and I remember feeling like I had peed my pants. At the time

I thought, "Oh, my water broke," but then I remembered my cervix was blocked, so it couldn't be my water and, as you probably have guessed, I looked down onto a pool of blood. I ran to the bathroom and sat on the toilet screaming at Luch to get my boots and jacket and keys and that we had to go to the hospital. The doctors had warned us that hemorrhaging was a risk factor and if bleeding started to happen to get the hospital ASAP. We luckily made it to our hospital within 30 minutes, which to this day I don't know how, because it was rush hour and we were dependent on the highway to get us there. After being checked into the hospital and set up with a monitor, the doctor quickly decided that there was no more time to waste and that they needed to get the baby out as I was in labour and at risk.

At 7:21 p.m., our little Brio was born. Liana Francisca Miranda weighed in at a tiny five pounds 13 ounces. Our little angel came out screaming. She had 10 toes and 10 fingers and she was the most beautiful sight I had ever seen: full head of hair, skinny little arms and legs—she was perfect. Everything in that moment was perfect, but then things started to get tense. The room became tense; Luch was asked to leave and things started to get scary. At the time that Luch was asked to leave, I was not too sure what was going on. I could hear the doctor telling the nurses to page the other OB on call, I could hear the anaesthetist calling down to the blood bank for units of blood and I could feel myself becoming anxious. The room went from a calm happy "We just had a baby" vibe to a room full of nurses, two surgeons and an anaesthetist assistant whose sole job was to hold my hand and keep me calm. My primary OB leaned down to me and said, "Sweetie, you have a condition that was undetected. Your placenta has formed into your uterus and we can't control your bleeding. We are prepping you for a hysterectomy." He kept asking me if I understood what it was that he was saying to me and I reassured him that I did. I believe my exact words were, "I have one baby—do what you need to do to save me."

During the time they were prepping me for my hysterectomy, I started to feel very different. I remember asking the anaesthetist if he was putting me under full anaesthesia— I felt as though an elephant was on my chest and I could not breathe. I started to get anxious and was yelling that I did not feel right and that I was feeling a pressure on my chest and a numbness rising up my body. The surgeon looked at the anaesthetist and I could hear him asking if it was possible that my spinal block could be moving up my spine. The anaesthetist answered no, and that is when, for the first time during the whole ordeal, I thought I might be dying. I had dealt with death before, but it was different when I was a cancer patient because my death was never imminent, it was something that could happen in a few months or years. This scenario—this was different. I could feel death right around the corner and I was so scared. I was alone in a room full of strangers; the scariest part of it all was that I had not even had the chance to touch my little Liana. How could I be dying without even having had the chance to feel her and tell her I love her?

Things started to happen very quickly; I had a whole team of nurses turn me on to my side, trying to get a plastic-like material under me, and the next thing I knew I was being wrapped in this plastic wrap and could feel hot air being pushed inside of it, getting me warm. When I was turned onto my side I was exposed to a scene of horror. Blood was everywhere—on the walls, on the ceiling, on the floor, on nurses scrubs—I was so confused. Why was there so much blood everywhere and how could my blood have ended up all over the place? I think one of the nurses must have seen the look of sheer panic in my eyes because she knelt on the floor beside me and very reassuringly said, "Honey, that was a bag of blood that burst as we were trying to get you hooked up to the transfusion pump." Thank goodness I thought. Back on my back, I was slowly feeling better; the weight had lifted off of my chest and I no longer felt as if I was crossing over to the other side. What I had experienced was hemorrhagic shock, or as I like to call it "WTF is happening to me" shock.

The next thing I remember is waking up in a surgical recovery room with my body still fully wrapped, and hot air being circulated in my wrap. I could not stop shaking or shivering; I was so scared. I had no idea what had happened, if I had a uterus or not, if my baby was okay…Where was Luch? I had so many questions.

After what felt like an eternity, Luch was by my side. He explained to me that doctors were able to get my bleeding under control and with some other measures, they were able to save my uterus. They were going to keep a close eye on me for the next 24 hours, but for the most part I seemed to be out of harm's way. That morning, sometime around 4:00 a.m., I held my baby girl for the first time. She was so small, so warm; our little Brio, she was perfection.

Having had some time to reflect on what happened to me, I am becoming more and more convinced that when it comes to medical odds or, should I say, things happening when the odds of them happening are so low, seems to be the way things just go with me. Why was it that all these rare occurrences seemed to be happening to me? How many times could I defy the odds and beat death? I don't have the answer to this. All I do know is that it's how I choose to walk away from these experiences that will shape my future and my outlook on life. My birthing experience has given me an even greater appreciation for life—not just my life, all life. The miracle of conception (whether it's natural or supported), the miracle of birth and survival—it's all an amazing gift that we must stop to appreciate and not take for granted. When life gets tough, which it does and the days get consumed with stress due to work or other things going on in your life, those are the moments to stop and reflect on what truly matters. Focus on the miracles, the ability to be alive, the miracle of life; focus on the good and the rest will settle into place.

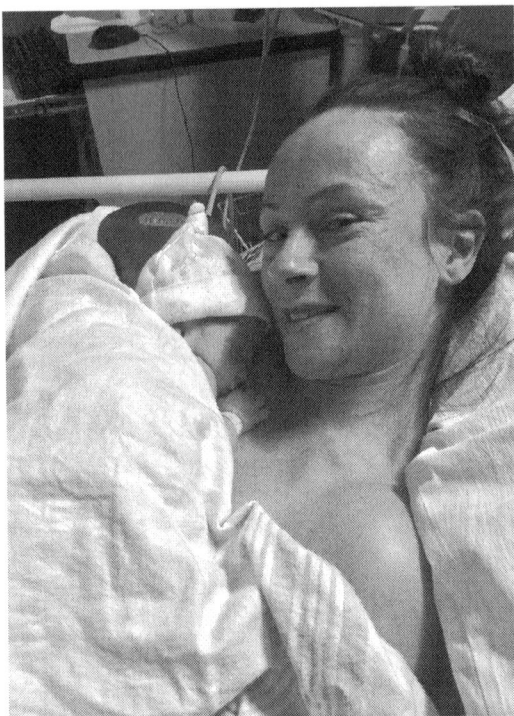

Me holding Liana for the first time

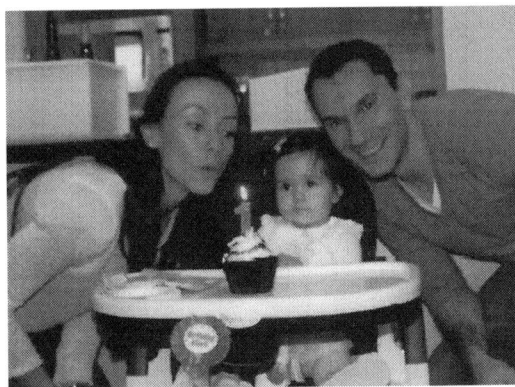

Luch and I helping Liana blow our her 1st birthday candle

12 #honouryourdays

Never in my wildest dreams could I ever have imagined that I would become a Reebok Ambassador in my mid-thirties. Let's recall that I was beyond shy as a kid growing up into my teens, and leading up to my early twenties I was very self-conscious. Post-cancer Lina was more confident and had a greater zest for life but still never would have imagined that she could become a brand ambassador for a leading sports apparel company. This just goes to show you that our futures can always hold some pretty unforeseen and wonderful surprises.

It was the late summer of 2015 and I was working from my home office. I remember feeling a bit of data paralysis, so I decided to take a break from my spreadsheet and check my personal email. After quickly scrolling through my emails I opened up a message from the gym where I teach my fitness classes. The email was forwarded to employees on behalf of Reebok Canada. Reebok Canada was running a contest looking for women whose lives had been changed through fitness. I distinctly remember closing the email and thinking "Why bother? There are probably other women with stories that are so much more compelling than mine." And right there, in that moment, I had a very significant DNA moment, because I was faced to walk the walk I preach to others and not be a fake. I'd always prided myself on challenging people to take risks and step outside of their comfort zones and, yet, here I was doing the exact thing that I always tell people to not do—doubt themselves. It was actually a very cathartic moment for me because it helped remind me that there are never any successes if chances are not taken. Yes, I would be setting myself up for possible rejection, but at the same time, I knew that if I didn't enter I would lose this potential opportunity to try and influence and help others through my story.

Weeks went by and it was radio silent: no responses, and no feedback. It was almost a month after my submission that I received an email from an ad agency that was hired to work on the 2016 campaign for Reebok. I was informed that I was chosen as one of the top 20 female finalists in Canada and they were requesting a Skype interview with me to review my story so that they could put together a profile of me which they would then pitch to Reebok. The marketing team at Reebok would then make the final decision which six women would be part of the 2016 campaign. I nearly fell off my chair with excitement; I couldn't believe that out of the hundreds of submissions they received, I had made it into the final 20.

The Skype interview happened about a week after my email response from the ad agency. I remember being so nervous for it. I contemplated for quite some time as to what to wear (Do I wear Reebok? Or would that be trying too hard? Makeup or no makeup?) I think I lost some sleep the night before trying to find the answers to my meaningless questions. I ended up wearing a simple T-shirt, hair down, no makeup. I figured that if I was going to be chosen it would be for my story and passion for fitness, not my choice of wardrobe or hairstyle.

The interview went really well. The gentleman that I was speaking to from the agency was super kind and very easy to talk to. He asked me questions about my childhood, my life before and after my illness, and how fitness changed my life. I became emotional in the interview and started to cry as I shared my story. I could not remember the last time I cried sharing my story, but for some reason on this day, my emotions were heightened. It was as though I was feeling them for the first time. I had shared many times with many people what my survival rate was and I how lucky and blessed I was to have survived. I had shared many times how my outlook on life had changed and how much I owed to fitness for changing me and allowing me to become the person that I am today, but it was as though I had never actually felt the emotions behind my words before because I broke down in this interview. I'm talking about actually having to step away from the computer and walk up and down the hallway to catch my breath breaking down. After managing to pull myself together, I walked back to the computer and apologized for losing control of my emotions and promised the guy I was talking to that I was not usually this emotional and that I could get myself together if I were chosen. The interview ended shortly after and I was told that I should hear back with their final decision within a few weeks.

The next few weeks felt like an eternity. I just wanted to know. I wanted to know if I could have the platform to share with others just how great the benefits of fitness are, to shed some rays of hope on others who have been told that they may not survive their illness; to provide perspective in times of despair. I wanted it really bad.

Two weeks later almost to the day, the email came and I was chosen!

Filming was scheduled to happen at my house a few months later. They were bringing a film crew to my condo to tape an interview and then they wanted to film me teaching a class at the gym. I remember waking up the morning of the filming feeling how I felt on Christmas Day when I was a kid. The crew showed up bright and early and they all managed to squeeze into our small condo. What amazed me was how everyone had an assistant. The cameraman, the lighting guy, the audio guy, the computer guy—everyone had a "someone" that helped them do their job. It was all so much fun to be a part of.

The interview took almost four hours. I was asked to talk about myself starting from childhood and leading up to the year of my diagnosis. The interview itself was exhausting and emotionally challenging, and it happened again, the waterworks. I broke down again for the second time in years, but I managed to get through the full interview and felt like I had run a marathon by the time it was done. It was exhausting. Who would have thought that talking about yourself for hours could be so draining? I had a short break after the interview and then we were off to the gym to film a class—or at least that was all I thought we were doing.

The day we filmed at the gym was super windy. Like really windy—so windy that there was a vacuum being created between the two front doors of the gym, making it very difficult to open the front door. One of the shots they wanted was of me walking up to the gym and opening the front door, which proved to be a very tasking action. I remember having to brace my core, squeeze my glutes and focus on using all my upper body strength to get the door open without it looking like I was struggling. The whole thing was a bit of an oxymoron: here I was filming a commercial for Reebok about how fitness changed my life and I was having trouble opening a door. At least I provided entertainment for the front desk staff working that day. Actually, they were more like my cheerleading squad and offered up cheers and jumps and smiles every time I opened that damn door.

Finally, after we got the perfect "door opening" shot, the film crew wanted me to go through the motions of teaching a class without any members actually in the class—a dry run so to speak—only I was teaching with full weights. By the time my actual class was set to begin, I was running on pure adrenaline, thank goodness, because I was exhausted. But the exhaustion was well worth it. Being on stage and teaching to my members a class that truly helped me through one of the most difficult times in my life and being filmed for a commercial that would share this journey with so many was such a fulfilling experience. There I was being recorded doing what I love to do in the hopes that I could inspire others to be drawn towards the benefits of fitness. For the first time in years, I felt like my purpose as post-cancer Lina was being fulfilled.

The commercial aired in January 2016 online, along with a commercial on television, which featured all six women in the campaign. The response was amazing, humbling and filled me with gratitude. I had many people reach out to me to share their struggles with cancer. Others reached out to share that I had inspired them to lead a more active lifestyle and that they were going to start exercising. Truly, I was humbled and fulfilled.

The success of the campaign led to the marketing team at Reebok Canada deciding to run a second campaign for their fall/winter season. I had the amazing opportunity to work on a second social media campaign, this one with the hashtag, #honouryourdays. The second campaign was geared at getting the message across that we all have a finite number of days and that we should make the most of them by honouring our bodies. This message resonated so much with me as I have always been, and continue to be, a strong believer that we must make the most of our time here on earth, as we never know when it will be taken from us.

The experience with Reebok Canada in 2016 brought everything full circle; it provided me with the motivation and confirmation that I was on the right path. I was fuelled with the passion to continue my journey in completing this book and in pursuing my quest to further help others find their ray of light during cloudy times. More than anything, my newly founded role with Reebok Canada further solidified my belief that no matter our past or our experiences, we do have the ability to change our futures and become what we want to be. Looking back to that day when I initially closed the email and made a quick decision to not submit my story will forever be a great learning moment for me. That DNA moment has helped me and will continue to help me in many of my future decisions when I doubt myself or question the outcome of a situation. Had I taken the easy way out and not made myself vulnerable to rejection, I would have lost out on such an incredible opportunity and journey. Anytime that I am faced with a decision that I am hesitant to move forward on based on my own self-imposed limitations or anxieties, I am reminded that if I don't try, I will never succeed. Learning from our DNA moments and allowing the teachings to help shape our futures positively vs. negatively can help you achieve anything that you allow yourself to be open to. Welcome change, challenge yourself and don't deny the uncomfortable. Be hopeful, be present and be aware.

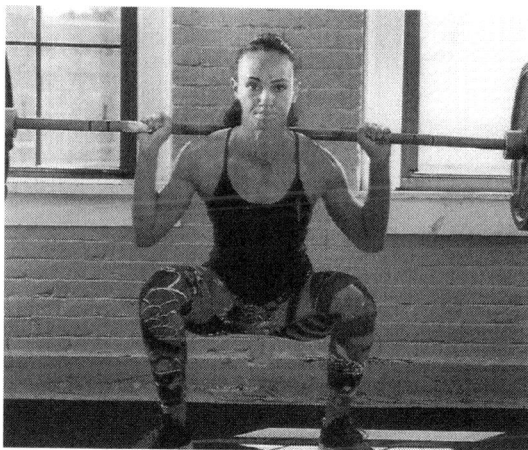

Pic from Reebok Canada's 2016
Honour Your Days campaign

13 Paradise

Like most people I really enjoy music: the energy that it can bring to any occasion and moment in life is magical at times. The appreciation that I have for the people that create music is immense. Artists have the ability to touch humans in such a unique manner. They have the power to get deep into our souls, tap into our emotions and bring to us the comfort or the energy that we seek from the music at that particular moment. Whether it's working out or sitting down to have dinner at home, music can set the mood and make the experience exponentially greater. Even more fascinating is the brain's natural ability to link music to our long-term memories. Hearing a song can instinctively take us back in time to a previous moment in our lives.

When I was going through my radiation treatments, I was allowed to; actually I was encouraged to bring music to my treatments. The radiation room was equipped with a sound system, speakers that would place music for the patients lying on the table. I used the same song for each one of my treatments, every 25 days. It was a trance song, no words, just beats, calming and hypnotic beats. For me, during those treatments of lying on a cold slab, having a machine move around me and shoot radiation to kill off my rogue cancer cells I was transported to a place where I felt warmth and peace and calmness, all through the beats of music that someone else had created. Now, whenever I hear that song, I am taken back to that very cold room where I was very sick and fighting for my life, but I'm not reminded about the dark moments, I am reminded of the comfort that the music brought me and I am reminded of how far I've come and how grateful I am to have survived.

One of my favourite soundtracks is from the movie *The Beach*, staring Leonardo DiCaprio. What I like in particular about this soundtrack is the variety of artists on the compilation and the mood that it puts me in; it takes me to my calm place. One of the songs on the soundtrack by Orbital has a very electronic feel to it and it features the voice of Leonardo DiCaprio. I quote, "Paradise…it's not where you go; it's how you feel for a moment in life and if you find it, it lasts forever." Oftentimes, we get caught up in our great search for this magical place or thing in life that will bring us happiness, a job, a new home, a new car; this constant struggle that we may find ourselves caught in and searching for can be exhausting and outright unhealthy for our well-being. If we can bring ourselves to the realization that paradise is not a place or a thing, but rather a feeling, then we can secure it and keep it forever.

When I started the journey of writing this book, I had a great deal of hesitation to work through. Self-doubt consumed me. I wondered why anyone would want to hear about my life and its various moments that stand out in my memory. However, now as I am approaching the end of this path, I am so grateful that I took the leap and dived into writing this book. Throughout my years as post-cancer

Lina, I have always tried to pride myself on providing my friends and family with solicited (and unsolicited) advice in the hopes of challenging them to dig deep and uncover the root of their actions. Challenging them to ask themselves what the motivation is that is driving their actions in question, and if their answer or conclusion makes them happy. My go-to reply is often, "If you were to find out tomorrow that you had a terminal or very debilitating illness, would you have no regrets about how you lived?" I hope I don't come across as a pessimist, because that is the furthest thing from what I want to be. My intent is to challenge people to make the decisions in life that will result in no regret. Having lived through a very difficult time and facing the reality of death, I know what it is like to have feelings of regret and wish that you would have done some things differently. To wish that you had not stressed over trivial things, to have not been so damn insecure, to have cared too much about what other people were thinking. To put it bluntly, it sucks, and when you're there, you make a promise to yourself to never to go back to that place.

We all have pasts; we all have had shitty things happen in our lives, for some shittier then others. We also have all had wonderful things happen to us. What makes you who you are is how you pave your future. So, how do you learn from your past experiences (good or bad) in order to shape your future? First and foremost, you must be honest with yourself. Accept your DNA moments; learn and grow from them. Take these moments that stand out in your memory and utilize them to understand yourself more deeply and allow yourself to reflect on how they may have moulded you into who you are today. If you are content with the outcome, awesome! But if you know that you are limiting your best version of you from surfacing because of an outcome, then make the change and empower yourself to become the person that you are proud of. You may not be able to change the past, but you are most definitely capable of shaping your future self.

Many of us may ask what our greater purpose in life is. Why has the greater being put us on this earth? I have spent countless nights laying awake in self-reflection trying to find an answer to this question, and for the first time in my life since post-cancer Lina was born, I can honestly and without a shred of doubt now say, my purpose is to help others make it over life's hurdles. I believe that in sharing the moments in my life that have helped shaped me into the person I am today, I may have an effect on someone else's life. My dream would be to be able to help as many people as I can to get through a tough time in their life or guide them through a decision or decisions. But in actuality, whether it's one person or 1000 people that I help, I feel like my purpose has been fulfilled.

I hope that I have inspired you to do some self-reflection, give some deeper thought to what has made you the person you are, by asking yourself why you choose or choose not to do the things that you do. Most important, I hope that you go on to find your paradise in life.

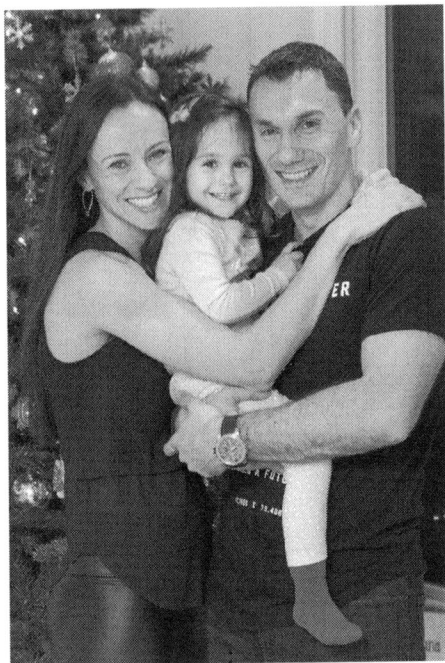

The 3 L's: Lina, Luch and Liana.

Made in the USA
Middletown, DE
06 November 2018

97578740R00083